Medicaid Financing Crisis:

BALANCING
RESPONSIBILITIES,
PRIORITIES,
AND DOLLARS

The Henry J. Kaiser Family Foundation

The Henry J. Kaiser Family Foundation was established by industrialist Henry J. Kaiser and his wife Bess in 1948 as an expression of their lifelong interest in medicine and their determination to improve health care. The Foundation is an independent philanthropy that focuses its grantmaking on the major health issues facing the nation, with a special interest in improving health and life chances of the disadvantaged. The Foundation is wholly separate from the Kaiser Permanente Medical Care Program and the Kaiser Industries, which Henry J. Kaiser also founded.

The Kaiser Commission on the Future of Medicaid

The Kaiser Commission on the Future of Medicaid was established by the Henry J. Kaiser Family Foundation in 1991 to function as a Medicaid policy institute and serve as a forum for analyzing, debating, and proposing future directions for program reform. Over the course of five years, the Commission will conduct analysis, convene meetings for policymakers, and issue fact-finding papers and policy reports with recommendations.

Medicaid Financing Crisis:

BALANCING
RESPONSIBILITIES,
PRIORITIES,
AND DOLLARS

Diane Rowland,
Judith Feder,
Alina Salganicoff, *editors*

The Kaiser Commission on the
Future of Medicaid

AAAS
PRESS

A publishing division of the American Association for the Advancement of Science

Library of Congress Cataloging-in-Publication Data

Medicaid financing crisis : balancing responsibilities, priorities, and
dollars / Diane Rowland, editor.
    p. cm. — (AAAS publication ; 93-04S)
    Commissioned by the Kaiser Commission on the Future of
Medicaid.
    Includes biographical references and index.
    ISBN 0-87168-514-0 (acid-free paper)
    1. Medicaid—Finance.   2. Insurance, Health—United States—
Finance.   3. Insurance, Health—Government policy—United States.
I. Rowland, Diane.   II. Kaiser Commission on the Future of
Medicaid.   III. Series.
    Q181.A1A8   no. 93-04S
    [HD7102.U]
    368.4'21'0973—dc20   93-11161
                                                 CIP

AAAS Publication: 93-04S
International Standard Book Number: 0-87168-514-0
Printed in the United States of America on acid-free paper

CONTENTS

•
•
•

Contents

LIST OF CONTRIBUTORS

•
•
•

Gerard Anderson, Ph.D., Director, Center for Hospital Finance and Management, The Johns Hopkins Medical Institutions, Baltimore, Maryland.

Gary J. Clarke, J.D., Assistant Secretary for Medicaid, Florida Health and Rehabilitative Services Department, Tallahassee, Florida.

Teresa Coughlin, M.P.H., Senior Research Associate, Urban Institute, Washington, DC.

Karen Davis, Ph.D., Executive Vice President, the Commonwealth Fund, New York, NY, and Chair, Financing Workgroup of the Kaiser Commission on the Future of Medicaid.

Judith Feder, Ph.D., Principal Deputy, Assistant Secretary, Planning and Evaluation, U.S. Department of Health and Human Services, Washington, DC; and formerly Associate Director of the Kaiser Commission on the Future of Medicaid.

Steven D. Gold, Ph.D., Director, Center for the Study of States, Nelson A. Rockefeller Institute of Government, Albany, New York.

David Heslam, Research Assistant, Urban Institute, Washington, DC.

John Holahan, Ph.D., Director, Health Policy Division, Urban Institute, Washington, DC.

Leighton Ku, Ph.D., Senior Research Associate, Urban Institute, Washington, DC.

Stephen H. Long, Ph.D., Senior Economist, The RAND Corporation, Washington, DC.

Victor J. Miller, Economic Management Consulting, Washington, DC.

Sara Rosenbaum, J.D., Senior Staff Scientist, The Center for Health Policy Research, The George Washington University, Washington, DC.

Diane Rowland, Sc.D., Executive Director, Kaiser Commission on the Future of Medicaid, Baltimore, Maryland.

Alina Salganicoff, Principal Policy Analyst, Kaiser Commission on the Future of Medicaid, Baltimore, Maryland.

William Scanlon, Ph.D., Co-Director, Center for Health Policy Studies, Georgetown University, Washington, DC.

Colin Winterbottom, Research Assistant, Urban Institute, Washington, DC.

ACKNOWLEDGMENTS

•
•
•

This book is the product of a collaborative effort of many individuals whose multiple contributions made this project a reality. We would like to express our heartfelt appreciation to the authors of this volume and are thankful for their ongoing research and analysis in Medicaid policy. Their continuing efforts will undoubtedly contribute to the resolution of the difficulties that the Medicaid program is currently confronting.

We would also like to extend our sincere appreciation to the Henry J. Kaiser Family Foundation, and particularly to Drew Altman and Dennis Beatrice, for their vision in establishing the Kaiser Commission on the Future of Medicaid and for their continuing support and guidance. We would also like to thank Matt James for his help in bringing this volume to fruition.

We are particularly thankful for the thoughtful comments and direction provided by the members of the Kaiser Commission on the Future of Medicaid, whose suggestions and deliberations contributed to the development of this volume. We would like to specifically thank James Tallon, the Commission's Chairman, and Karen Davis, Chair of the Commission's Financing Workgroup, who shaped our thinking in this area.

We cannot forget the contributions of the participants of the July 1992 roundtable discussion on the Medicaid financing crisis. Their thoughtful insights and comments were the genesis for the Kaiser Commission's subsequent analysis of the factors underlying the Medicaid spending growth.

A number of people have provided invaluable assistance in the production of this book. Special appreciation goes to Amanda McCloskey of the Commission staff for her critical role throughout the entire review and publication process. We are indebted to Louise R. Goines and other staff at AAAS Press, and to Nancy Lee Moran, copyeditor, for their guidance and perseverance throughout the chapter review and publication process.

Diana Rowland, Sc.D.
Judith Feder, Ph.D.
Alina Salganicoff

INTRODUCTION

JUDITH FEDER

•
•
•

In a health care system beleaguered with problems, Medicaid stands out as a program in crisis. Alongside widespread concern about limits to Medicaid's protection—the millions of low-income Americans the program fails to cover and the limited access to service for the millions it does cover—is shock at recent increases in Medicaid costs. With rates of increase at 19 percent in 1990 and 26 percent in 1991, Medicaid has gained an image as the "Pac Man"® of both state and federal budgets. Such rapid cost increases raise questions about state and federal governments' willingness and ability to sustain current program commitments, let alone proceed to expansion.

To better understand the implications of recent experience for future policy, the Kaiser Commission on the Future of Medicaid commissioned the seven chapters comprising this volume, which explore the following issues:

■ Why and how Medicaid costs have risen in recent years;

■ How cost increases reflect two fundamental policy issues—population coverage and provider payment; and

■ What recent cost increases imply for sharing fiscal responsibilities between federal and state governments.

A brief overview follows, summarizing each author's answers to these questions.

NATURE AND CAUSES OF SPENDING INCREASES

Stephen Long provides the context for this consideration of Medicaid costs by analyzing the history of Medicaid cost experience, the way in which the last two years have deviated from that history, and key factors contributing to that deviation.

Long's historical look at expenditures indicates that from 1980 through 1988, Medicaid spending increased at rates comparable to rates of increase for private insurance and Medicare. Spending increases in this period had little to do with increases in the population served. Instead, rising cost per beneficiary explained the bulk of the growth.

From 1988 through 1991, Medicaid grew at successively greater rates of 13, 19, and 26 percent—significantly faster than its historical trend of about 10 percent per year. Explaining the "excess" over the historical average, Long finds that expanded enrollment has contributed significantly in every year (at especially high levels in 1990 and 1991). Higher cost per beneficiary became a major factor in spending increases in 1991, when it explained half of the full 7-point increase in the spending growth rate over the previous year.

Long attributes somewhat less than half of the "excess" spending to enrollment increases due to the federal mandates for coverage of pregnant women and children. The remainder, in part, reflects increases in Aid to Families with Dependent Children (AFDC) enrollment that may be due to the recession. However, Long argues that other factors may be equally important to welfare expansions. State initiatives to promote program participation, through simplified eligibility processes or outreach efforts, may have increased not only Medicaid enrollment but also enrollment in the basic welfare programs, AFDC and Food Stamps.

With regard to cost increases, it becomes more difficult to assign causality to specific policies. Reliance on provider-specific taxes, voluntary contributions, and other financing mechanisms provided the states a previously untapped revenue source that facilitated both increases in beneficiaries and in costs per beneficiary. The latter increases in large part reflected higher payments to hospitals, as the states responded to legal pressure to comply with the Boren Amendment, which requires Medicaid to pay "the costs of efficiently and economically operated" institutions.

John Holahan and his coauthors draw on discussions with Medicaid officials and other public and private participants in Medicaid policy in nine states to bring to life the way the states themselves perceive the factors causing expenditures to rise. The Urban Institute team visited nine states, selected to include the largest of Medicaid programs, to provide a geographic spread and to reflect differences in circumstances (relatively restrictive eligibility standards; particularly harsh economic conditions) likely to affect their Medicaid programs.

Looking first at factors affecting enrollment, Holahan and his coauthors find that states identify mandates for pregnant women and children and the recession as primary sources of expansions. Not surprisingly, the states with initially restrictive eligibility (South Carolina, Texas, and, to a lesser extent, Florida and Missouri) emphasize the impact of the coverage mandate, noting, however, that it reflected their own objectives as much as federal law. The impact of the recession was more widely felt, but was particularly striking in the northeast and in California. Although some states attributed enrollment increases to mandates related to low-income elderly and, in California, to undocumented aliens, for the most part the states visited did not feel mandates other than those affecting pregnant women and children had been a major source of expansionary pressure. Furthermore, when asked specifically about pressure from AIDS, drug abuse, homelessness, or other social problems, the states perceived little direct impact.

Looking beyond enrollment, the states consistently identified pressure to keep up with cost inflation in the broader medical market as a major source of expenditure increases. Threat of litigation under the Boren Amendment by hospitals and nursing homes, limited control over prescription drug prices (despite recent legislation on rebates), and efforts to ensure access to the obstetric care so many Medicaid recipients need inhibit state efforts to limit what they pay. In addition, although the states have successfully constrained growth in institutional long-term care spending, home health care for the elderly and nonelderly disabled has become the fastest growing Medicaid benefit.

What Holahan and his coauthors found most striking in their interviews was the increasing aggressiveness with which the states have turned to Medicaid and its federal funds as a means to mitigate budgetary pressures, fend off cuts, or support program expansions at minimal state expense. Whether the mechanism was a shift to Medicaid from a state-funded program (for the mentally ill, the mentally retarded, maternal and child health, or other populations), reliance on provider-specific taxes and donations, or special payments to hospitals serving a "disproportionate share" of Medicaid and other low-income patients, the strategy and outcome was intentional and consistent—expanded access to federal funds to support not only Medicaid but overall care to the poor.

EXPANDING ACCESS AND PAYING PROVIDERS

Underlying the myriad of policies and circumstances that explain recent increases in Medicaid spending are the continuing pressures of covering the population in need and paying providers adequately to ensure access to care. Two chapters explore these fundamental issues, focusing on specific recent actions affecting each—federal mandates regarding scope of coverage (and, to a lesser extent, benefits and payment) and litigation based on the Boren Amendment regarding the adequacy of provider payment.

Sara Rosenbaum's assessment of several significant federally mandated Medicaid expansions between 1984 and 1990 illustrates both the importance of coverage to beneficiaries and the issues the states face in implementing coverage expansions. Starting with expanded coverage for pregnant women and children, Rosenbaum notes the "unprecedented" speed with which states implemented the expansions, a reflection of the states' support for these reforms. By 1991, more than half of all states exceeded minimum eligibility requirements for pregnant women and infants; 17 were at the minimum; and 47 states and the District of Columbia had eliminated asset tests as an eligibility requirement. In terms of people, estimates are that as many as 45 percent of all births in the United States may now be eligible for Medicaid coverage. Despite some limitations with respect to early enrollment of pregnant women and of older children, Rosenbaum emphasizes how important Medicaid has become to the nation's children, with its enhanced responsibility not only for coverage but for benefit content and provider settings that are most appropriate for children's needs.

Other expansions have been more problematic. As Rosenbaum reviews the intentions and effects of reforms, she illustrates a variety of complexities and conflicts that surround expansions. These include logistical problems and confusion about who bears the costs in reforms to facilitate enrollment; complexities, delivery problems, and potential costs in moving Medicaid into overseeing sufficient "content of care" in Early and Periodic Screening, Diagnosis, and Treatment (EPSDT) Program requirements; barriers to enrollment in requirements that Medicaid supplement Medicare for low-income seniors; and conflicts about the appropriate role of Medicaid and federal grant programs and the best way to pay for and manage care in the payment mandates for federally qualified health centers. While noting the potential value of these varied reforms to those who obtain better coverage and payment, Rosenbaum emphasizes the difficulties facing any expansions in a program fraught with controversy over who should pay.

The chapter by Gerard Anderson and William Scanlon examines issues related to determining reimbursement levels for Medicaid services—an issue that increasingly adds the conflict of litigation to the ever-present Medicaid institutional conflict between federal and state governments and the fundamental conflict in health care financing between controlling costs and ensuring access to care. Anderson and Scanlon explain how the vagueness of federal requirements for Medicaid payments to hospitals and nursing homes is involving the courts in critical policy decisions on payment. Court decisions are raising both procedural and substantive questions about state payment policy, are pressing the states to undertake extensive and burdensome analyses to defend their rates, and are inhibiting what may be inherently reasonable efforts to limit payments to providers. Anderson and Scanlon argue that the process of litigation should be replaced with a more systematic approach to payment oversight, whether through greater federal control, clearer federal standards, state-defined "all-payer" systems, or other means.

FEDERAL AND STATE ROLES IN FINANCING

The final three chapters shift our focus from how Medicaid spends its dollars to where it gets the dollars—in particular, to the struggle between federal and state governments and the burdens on both that Medicaid financing increasingly represents.

Victor Miller examines Medicaid in the context of federal grants-in-aid, documenting the way cuts in other federal grant programs and changes in the federal budgeting process dramatically increased the importance of Medicaid to the states as a source of federal funds. These shifts, which began in the early 1980s and accelerated thereafter, are reversing the previous decline in federal grants to state and local governments, increasing Medicaid's share of grants from 21 percent in 1985 to 42 percent in 1993. In the last few years, higher Medicaid matching rates for most states (reflecting variation in income growth across states) and a variety of financing devices (provider-specific taxes and donations and intergovernmental transfers) helped many states weather the fiscal and program pressures created by the recession, program mandates, and other factors. Using Health Care Financing Administration data, Miller reports that states used financing devices for $6.9 billion in state matching funds to generate $11 billion in federal funds in 1992. Of the total spending increase attributed to states between 1991 and 1992, three eighths actually involved no general-fund state revenues.

Miller raises some questions about the desirability and sustainability of recent financing strategies. First, the new rules on allowable practices leave considerable room for executive discretion at both the state and federal levels, with controversy, inconsistency, and lack of legislative oversight likely to result. In his view, the rules may become unworkable. Second, and perhaps more significant in the long run, Miller argues that, absent health care reforms, federal budget reforms in the next Congress will limit the states' capacity to draw on federal funds. Such actions would return to the states greater fiscal responsibility for managing their Medicaid spending.

Steven Gold assesses the states' capacity to handle that responsibility with an examination of Medicaid's place in state budgets. Arguing that the best measure of Medicaid's fiscal burden is at the margin, Gold points to estimates that the 1991–1992 increase in state Medicaid appropriations absorbed close to half the total increase in state appropriations in that year. Medicaid is now the fastest growing category of state spending, surpassing corrections in the last few years. Sizable increases in spending in these categories (and, in response to enrollment increases, in elementary and secondary education) have come to some extent at the expense of increases in other categories. Last year, many states actually cut welfare benefits and spending for higher education.

The states' capacity to spend depends, of course, on their capacity to raise revenues. Although state and local taxes are today a smaller proportion of income than they were in the 1970s, taxes have risen faster than income over the past decade. Gold expects that taxes, along with user charges, will continue to rise in the future. However, with incomes stagnant, he believes revenue growth will be insufficient to support high priority improvements in infrastructure, social services, and higher education. Gold emphasizes that states vary considerably in their "tax effort" or willingness to tax available resources, as well as in the resources that constitute "tax capacity." Given such variation, he concludes that reliance on the states to finance Medicaid will inevitably mean variation not only in the program's adequacy across states, but also in the extent to which Medicaid's adequacy comes at other programs' expense.

Gary Clarke draws on his experience managing Medicaid in Florida to challenge whether such extensive reliance on states to finance Medicaid or broader care to the poor makes sense. Emphasizing his own and other states' innovations in facilitating program participation, reaching populations with special needs, processing claims, and, perhaps most important, promoting effective service delivery, Clarke argues there is nothing fundamentally wrong with the states' ability to manage their Medicaid programs. The problem, he believes, is that states lack the resources to finance these programs.

In Clarke's view, future Medicaid policy should distinguish program management from program financing. State governments should continue to design and to operate programs tailored to their citizens' particular needs and sustain current contributions to program costs. But fiscal responsibility for covering the new populations, broader benefits, and higher service costs that adequate coverage requires should rest with the federal government, which has the means to pay for it.

Taken together, the chapters in this book provide a comprehensive picture of the fundamental policy issues underlying the Medicaid crisis. These chapters were initially Commission-sponsored papers prepared for the Commission's roundtable discussion, "The Medicaid Financing Crisis: Balancing Responsibilities, Priorities, and Dollars," in July 1992. The purpose of the roundtable was to discuss the findings from the Commission-sponsored research on the factors underlying the recent Medicaid cost increases and financing problems, as well as to explore the implications of these findings on current and future policy. To obtain multiple perspectives on the causes of the escalating cost growth, the Commission invited federal and state legislative and executive officials and health policy analysts to participate in the roundtable discussion. The highlights of the discussion are summarized in this volume by Karen Davis, chair of the Commission's financing workgroup.

Following the roundtable discussion, the Commission contracted with the Urban Institute to conduct an analysis to assess the relative roles of the factors contributing to Medicaid spending increases from 1988 to 1991. Specifically, the Commission requested that the Urban Institute disaggregate the impact of enrollment growth from increases in prices and use. The findings of that research are presented in the Kaiser Commission on the Future of Medicaid report, *The Medicaid Cost Explosion: Causes and Consequences,* and are summarized at the conclusion of this volume in the epilogue by Rowland and Salganicoff.

The Commission hopes that the information furnished by the chapters of this volume will begin to establish the foundation of knowledge necessary to build recommendations for future reform and strengthen the health financing and delivery systems to better serve the poor and vulnerable of this country.

PART 1

• • •

Nature and Causes of Spending Increases

•

Causes of Soaring Medicaid Spending, 1988–1991

STEPHEN H. LONG

INTRODUCTION

During the last three years Medicaid spending has soared, whether measured against previous trends in its own spending, or against past and current trends in public and private health care spending. Data from the Health Care Financing Administration (HCFA) form 64s and budget estimates show that the recent increases have transformed a roughly $50 billion program in 1987 to one exceeding $90 billion in 1991 (see Figure 1).

Medicaid grew at reasonably steady rates of about 10 percent per year through most of the 1980s. But then its rate of annual increase rose steadily to 13 percent in 1989, 19 percent in 1990, and 26 percent in 1991 (see Figure 2).

Historically, Medicaid has been the smallest of the three major types of health insurance in the United States, spending less than private insurance and Medicare (see Figure 3). Through much of its history, the growth of total Medicaid spending has been in line with that for other health insurance programs. For example, from 1980 through 1988, the average an-

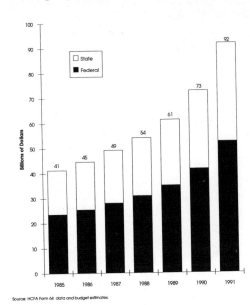

Source: HCFA Form 64 data and budget estimates.

Figure 1. Growth in Absolute Medicaid Spending, 1985–1991.

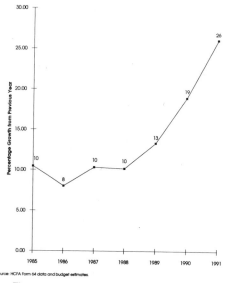

Figure 2. Relative Growth in Medicaid Spending, 1985–1991.

nual rate of growth for each program was between 10 and 11 percent. In contrast, the latest federal projections, based in part on rapid current growth, show Medicaid's growth rate at about double those of the other programs between 1988 and 1995 (see Figure 4). These trends imply that Medicaid spending will overtake that of Medicare by 1993 (Figure 3).

Illustrative of the alarm this new trend caused at the federal level was the formation of an interagency "SWAT team" in 1991 by Office of Management and Budget (OMB) Director Richard Darman, to explore the causes of Medicaid spending growth. In 1992, when announcing his health reform proposal, former President Bush declared that the federal government must get its health care spending under control. To make his point, he cited that in 1992 alone Medicaid spending was expected to increase by 38 percent. Coincident with this growing federal concern, the states are increasingly hard-pressed to find revenues to meet their share of the rising expenditures for Medicaid, one of the fastest growing elements in their budgets.

Figure 3. Actual and Projected Spending for Major Third-Party Payers.

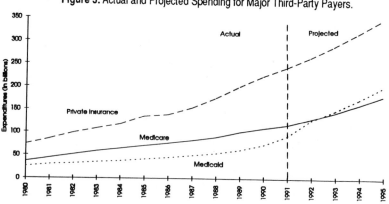

Source: HCFA, Office of the Actuary, and Administration budget estimates, various years.

Medicaid has clearly become a major fiscal concern for both federal and state government payors. To understand the fiscal pressures that will shape Medicaid's future requires further examination of historical and projected spending growth and factors contributing to that growth. Beginning by enumerating the most common hypotheses about the causes of the recent spending surge, and then making use of recently available data for 1991, this chapter attempts to measure the relative contributions of these various causes to the overall growth.

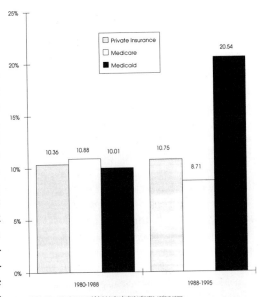

Source: HCFA, Office of the Actuary, and Administration budget estimates, various years.

Figure 4. Rate of Growth of Actual and Projected Spending for Major Third-Party Payers.

HYPOTHESES

There are many hypotheses put forth about the causes of the recent surge in Medicaid spending. Some suggest reasons why the number of beneficiaries would grow, while others would lead to increases in payments per beneficiary. Both would contribute to overall spending increases.

The following factors could be contributing to increased costs as a result of *increased numbers of beneficiaries:*

- The federal mandates of the 1980s have led to increased eligibility among both pregnant women and infants; and

- The recession has caused increased enrollment in the Aid to Families with Dependent Children (AFDC) program, thereby increasing the number of Medicaid eligibles.

The following factors could be contributing to *increased spending per beneficiary:*

- Provider payment rates may be rising faster than they would have otherwise due to the threat of or the success of Boren Amendment lawsuits over hospital and nursing home payment levels; and

- Providers may be receiving greater payments funded by provider tax and donation programs.

BASELINE TRENDS, 1980–1988

Examining the components of expenditure growth provides insight into the forces shaping those expenditures. The simplest approach is to "decompose" the annual rate of growth into the product of the rate of growth in the number of beneficiaries and the rate of growth in the cost per beneficiary.

Medicaid expenditures between 1980 and 1988 grew at an average annual rate of 10 percent (Figure 2). Growth in the number of Medicaid beneficiaries during this period, from 21.6 million to 22.9 million, explains only a small amount of the growth in expenditures. The number of Medicaid beneficiaries grew at an average annual rate of only 0.8 percent. The growth rate for disabled beneficiaries was somewhat higher than the average, but the number of elderly beneficiaries declined over this period. Taken together, disabled and elderly beneficiaries accounted for about 20 percent of the 1.3 million added beneficiaries, while AFDC beneficiaries accounted for about 80 percent of that number.

Most of the historical growth in Medicaid spending can be attributed either to price increases for the medical and long-term care services it purchased on behalf of beneficiaries or to other factors such as utilization increases. There are no good direct annual measures of these factors. Provider reimbursement increases in Medicaid almost surely fell below their rate of increase in other programs. Less is known about utilization changes.

To measure the contributions of the above factors toward program spending, and to provide a forecasting tool to predict what would have happened to spending in the absence of the hypothesized changes above, an econometric model of spending was estimated using data for 1980 through 1988. The model estimates the relationship between total Medicaid spending and two independent variables—the total number of Medicaid beneficiaries and the level of the Medical Care component of the Consumer Price Index (MCCPI). This latter variable serves as a proxy for the combined effect of payment policy and utilization levels—that is, factors affecting the cost per beneficiary. The model and the data to which it was fitted are described in detail in the Appendix at the end of this chapter.

Figure 5 shows three spending patterns for 1980 to 1991. The first is actual Medicaid spending in all years. The second is the model fit to the historical data for 1980 through 1988, and then predicted using the actual post-1988 levels of Medicaid enrollment and medical prices. The similarity between actual spending and this prediction reflects the effectiveness of the model in tracking the impact of major enrollment shifts. The third pattern is similar to the second, but it assumes the 1980–1988 trend in enrollment growth had persisted. This last pattern, which would have led to considerably lower spending by 1991, represents the baseline used in this paper.

This particular use of the term "baseline" merits some discussion. Its purpose is to allow a basic distinction to be made between two paths of

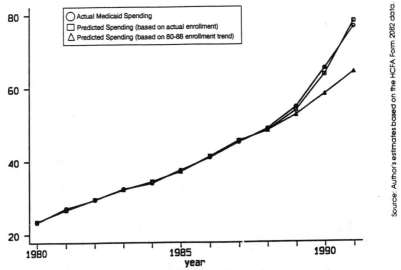

Figure 5. Actual and Estimated Medicaid Spending Under Alternative Enrollment Assumptions.

Medicaid spending between 1988 and 1991: (1) what would have happened had the enrollment trends of 1980–1988 and the prior relationship between medical prices and Medicaid spending persisted—the baseline; and (2) the additional impact of planned as well and unplanned enrollment growth plus any additional influences on the cost per beneficiary. This usage is different from the concept of baseline for budget estimates, where the enrollment growth from current law would be included as part of the baseline.

CAUSES OF GROWTH IN ADDITION TO BASELINE TRENDS, 1988–1991

Figure 6 summarizes the principal findings of this study. Most of the 1989, 1990, and 1991 spending increases in addition to baseline trends can be attributed to the unprecedented growth in Medicaid enrollment, especially in 1990 and 1991. Moreover, by 1991 the first signs of the influence of payment increases financed by provider taxes and donations became apparent, although their full effect is unlikely to appear until 1992.

As discussed earlier, the 1980–1988 trend was a 10 percent annual growth in total Medicaid spending. This can be "decomposed" into roughly a 1 percentage point increase in spending due to enrollment growth and a residual increase in the spending per beneficiary of about 9 percentage points, depending on the exact rate of medical price inflation.

In 1989 spending grew by approximately 13 percent. This increase may be allocated to four causes. First, the increase that would have occurred if enrollment grew at its 1980–1988 rate is about 1 percentage point. Second,

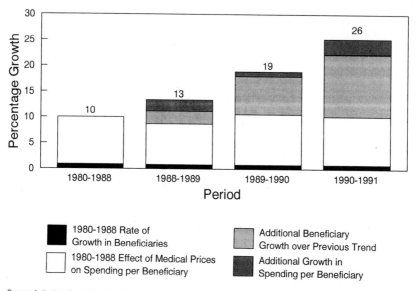

Source: Author's estimates based on the HCFA Form 2082 data, Form 64 data, and budget reports.

Figure 6. Factors Contributing to Recent Medicaid Spending Growth.

the increase arising from the effect of that year's medical price inflation (as a proxy for several factors) on spending per beneficiary is about 8 percentage points. Next, the increase attributable to the excess growth in the number of beneficiaries over and above the previous trend accounts for about 2.5 percentage points. Finally, the residual increase from greater spending per beneficiary than expected from the effect of medical price increases alone represents about 2 percentage points.

The 1990 rate of 19 percent and the 1991 rate of 26 percent may be allocated in an analogous fashion. Baseline enrollment and cost per beneficiary account for about 10.5 percentage points of the totals in each year. Also, in 1990 the additional beneficiary growth of about 1.6 million people (a 6.6 percent increase) accounts for about 7 percentage points of the remaining 8.5 percentage points of spending growth. Aside from being much larger than in previous years, the result for 1991 is similar. The 2.8 million additional enrollees account for about 12 of the 16 percentage points of "additional" growth above baseline. There remains about a 4 percentage point increase in cost per beneficiary.

To restate the 1991 results in dollars, total spending grew by $19 billion, from $73 billion to $92 billion (Figure 1). Of this $19 billion growth, $7.5 billion would have happened had the 1980 to 1988 trends prevailed. About $9 billion of the additional spending is estimated to be a result of additional beneficiaries served, many of them because of legislated eligibility expansions. There was a residual increase of roughly $2.5 billion in the cost per beneficiary.

Number of Beneficiaries

The total number of Medicaid beneficiaries has been expanding rapidly since 1989. According to HCFA data, total beneficiaries grew from 23.5 million to 25.3 million, or 7.4 percent, between 1989 and 1990. They rose again in 1991 to 28.3 million, for a change of 3.0 million, or nearly 12 percent.

Table 1 shows the 1991 data on beneficiary increases disaggregated by reason of eligibility. Just under one half, or 1.46 million, of the new beneficiaries were reported as qualifying under the provisions of recent legislation, consistent with the "federal mandates" hypothesis. Another 30 percent, or 860,000, of the additional beneficiaries were eligible for Medicaid by virtue of receiving some form of cash assistance, which is consistent with the "recession-induced" hypothesis.

Table 1. Change in Medicaid Beneficiaries by Assistance Status, 1990–1991.

Assistance Status	1991 Beneficiaries (in thousands)	1990–1991 Change (in thousands)	1990–1991 Percent Change
TOTAL	28,258	3,003	12
Cash	17,327	859	5
Non-Cash and Medically Needy	7,293	700	11
Recent Legislation	3,541	1,462	70
AFDC	20,758	2,538	14
Cash	12,779	653	5
Non-Cash and Medically Needy	5,309	720	16
Recent Legislation	2,670	1,165	78
AGED	3,353	151	5
Cash	1,502	−24	−2
Non-Cash and Medically Needy	1,263	−15	−1
Recent Legislation	588	189	47
DISABLED	4,051	333	9
Cash	3,046	229	8
Non-Cash and Medically Needy	720	−5	−1
Recent Legislation	284	109	62

Source: HCFA Forms 2082, 1990 and 1991.

From the perspective of assistance categories, 84 percent of the enrollment growth was in the AFDC category. Of the new enrollees, just under half became eligible through recent legislation, about one quarter also receive cash assistance, and the remaining are reported to be in traditional Medic-aid-only groups. The remaining 16 percent of the growth came from the disabled (11 percent) and the aged (5 percent). This mix is similar to the 80 percent/20 percent split of AFDC and disabled in the 1980–1988 period.

What does this mix of new beneficiaries imply about their costs? Unfortunately, the available data do not provide a direct measure of the additional beneficiaries' costs. If we assume that the within-group average cost is the same for former and new beneficiaries, however—that is, only the proportions of eligibility groups vary—then the average cost of the newly enrolled would be $2,075, or about 75 percent of the cost for the average Medicaid beneficiary. The fact that the AFDC adults are more likely to be pregnant could raise this estimate to about 80 percent. This estimate based on the mix of new beneficiaries is somewhat lower than the assumption in our econometric model. Based on historical experience, it was estimated that the additional enrollees cost about the same as existing ones (see Appendix). This is clearly a subject for further research.

Are the hypotheses stated at the outset of this paper that implied growth in beneficiaries supported by the data? The role of federal mandates and options for covering pregnant women and children is clearly supported by the data. The observation that the number of adults and children from low-income families receiving AFDC would grow is consistent with the recession-induced hypothesis.

To further explore the recession-induced hypothesis, trends in AFDC enrollments and the number of unemployed between 1985 and 1991 were examined (see Figure 7). Although AFDC enrollments have risen recently, as have the numbers of unemployed, examination of the entire period raises concern about whether a causal relationship can be concluded. The AFDC figures were relatively steady, at about 11 million enrollees from the winter of 1984–1985 through the fall of 1989. Then they rose rapidly to 11.6 million

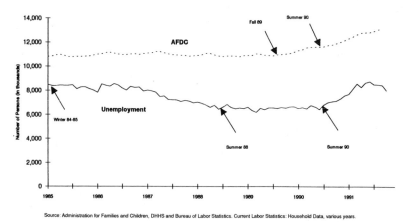

Source: Administration for Families and Children, DHHS and Bureau of Labor Statistics. Current Labor Statistics: Household Data, various years.

Figure 7. Unemployment and AFDC Enrollment, 1985–1991.

Table 2. Medicaid funding programs that utilize voluntary contributions and provider taxes, 1991.

	Type of Program		Dollars (in millions)			% of State Share*	Source of Funds						
	Tax	Donation	State	Federal	Total		Hospital	Nursing Home	Physic.	Pharm.	DSH	Expand Eligibility	Other
California		x	65	65	130	2	x		x		x	x	
Florida	x	x	158	189	347	11					x	x	x
Georgia		x	36	58	94	5	x				x	x	
Kentucky	x		59	158	217	15	x	x	x	x	x	x	x
Maine	x(2)		2	2	4	1	x						x
Maryland	x	x	34	34	68	5	x	x	x	x			x
Michigan		x	401	498	899	30	x	x					x
Missouri		x	80	124	204	16	x					x	x
New Jersey	x		8	8	16	1	x						
New York	x		148	148	296	2	x	x	x	x			x
North Carolina		x	53	105	158	8	x				x		x
Ohio	x		38	59	97	2	x				x		
Pennslyvania		x	515	678	1193	28	x	x			x		x
South Carolina	x	x	9	24	33	3	x	x				x	x
Tennessee	x		68	147	215	11	x	x				x	x
Utah		x	5	15	20	6	x	x			x		x
TOTAL or MEAN**	10	10	$1,679	$2,312	$3,991	9	15	8	4	3	8	7	12

*Percent of state share is based on the state portion of taxes and donations as a percent of the total state share of Medicaid expenditures.

**All figures are totals except "percent of state share," which is an unweighted mean.

Source: Tabulations based on data from "Voluntary Contributions and Provider Specific Taxes Survey Results." American Public Welfare Association, July and August 1991.

Table 3. Medicaid funding programs that utilize voluntary contributions and provider taxes, 1992.

	Type of Program		Dollars (in millions)			% State Share*	Source of Funds				Use of Funds		
	Tax	Donation	State	Federal	Total		Hospital	Nursing Home	Physic.	Pharm.	DSH	Expand Eligibility	Other
Alabama	x		174	464	638	40	x	x		x	x	x	x
Arkansas	x	x	30	91	121	15							x
California		x	65	65	130	1	x	x	x	x	x	x	x
Florida	x	x	259	310	569	14	x				x	x	x
Georgia		x	88	139	227	10	x				x	x	
Illinois	x		640	640	1280	35	x				x	x	
Indiana	x		60	105	165	8	x	x			x		x
Kentucky	x		157	423	580	35	x				x	x	x
Maine	x(2)		85	148	233	27	x	x				x	x
Maryland	x	x	143	143	286	18	x		x	x			x
Michigan		x	452	534	986	37	x	x	x	x			
Minnesota	x		51	59	110	5	x				x		
Mississippi	x	x	59	235	294	23	x	x		x			x
Missouri		x	160	238	398	38	x	x			x		x
Montana	x		2	4	6	2							x
Nevada	x		25	25	50	20		x	x	x			x
New Hampshire	x		35	35	70	16	x						x
New Jersey	x		8	8	16	1	x				x		
New York	x		200	200	400	3	x		x	x		x	
North Carolina		x	67	134	201	11	x	x	x		x		x
Ohio	x		44	67	111	3	x				x		x
Pennsylvania		x	565	738	1303	28	x						x
South Carolina	x	x	124	328	452	63	x	x				x	x
Tennessee	x		344	750	1094	46	x	x			x	x	x
Utah		x	5	16	21	5	x	x				x	x
Vermont	x		7	11	18	12	x	x			x		x
Washington	x		30	35	65	7	x	x			x		x
Wisconsin	x		16	25	41	2	x	x			x		x
TOTAL or MEAN**	21	11	$3,895	$5,970	$9,864	19	25	15	7	7	16	10	21

*Percent of state share is based on the state portion of taxes and donations as a percent of the total state share of Medicaid expenditures.

**All figures are totals except "percent of state share," which is an unweighted mean.

Source: Tabulations based on data from "Voluntary Contributions and Provider Specific Taxes Survey Results." American Public Welfare Association, July and August 1991.

by the summer of 1990. But from the summer of 1988 through the summer of 1990, the unemployment rate did not vary by more than 0.2 percentage points—it stayed between 5.2 and 5.4 percent of the labor force, or about 6.5 million people. So the rapid rise in AFDC enrollments, beginning in late 1989, preceded the rise in unemployment, starting in mid-1990, by at least six months!

This evidence suggests that the continuing rise in AFDC enrollments through 1991, which had the effect of increasing Medicaid eligibility, has at least one other cause besides the recession. It also suggests that the rise in eligibility may not fall off during a forthcoming economic recovery. There was no such effect on AFDC enrollments between January 1985 and summer 1988 when the unemployment rate fell by 2 percentage points, or about 2 million people (see Figure 7).

The growth in AFDC enrollment appears to bring increased Medicaid eligibles, but its sole cause does not appear to be the recession. There has been some speculation that the "outreach" efforts of the states to attract newly eligible pregnant women may have increased participation rates among those who are eli-

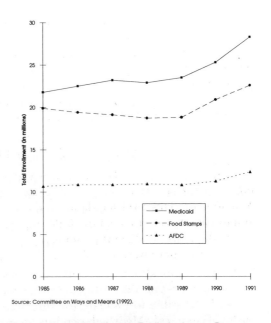

Source: Committee on Ways and Means (1992).

Figure 8. Annual Enrollment in Public Assistance Programs, 1985–1991.

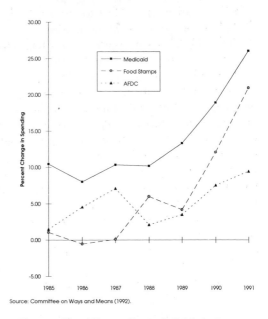

Source: Committee on Ways and Means (1992).

Figure 9. Annual Percent Change in Public Assistance Programs Spending, 1985–1991.

13

gible for AFDC cash assistance and, therefore, Medicaid. This effect has not been quantified. It is consistent with evidence on trends in enrollment and spending in three major public assistance programs, however. Figures 8 and 9 show that the "takeoff" in Medicaid enrollment and spending starting in 1989 was accompanied by similar trends in AFDC and in Food Stamps. There is a serious need to better understand the causes of this relatively abrupt and simultaneous growth among programs.

Increases in Provider Payments

One commonly cited reason why states' provider payments are increasing faster of late is vigorous enforcement in the courts of the Boren Amendment. This 1981 legislation requires states' payments to hospitals and nursing homes to meet the following test: They must, at a minimum, cover "the costs of efficiently and economically operated facilities." As of July 1, 1991, there were lawsuits over Medicaid hospital payments in 12 states (1). It is not known in how many other states the possibility or threat of legal action is causing more generous payment policies to be undertaken. It may be possible to estimate the direct contribution of court-ordered payment changes to Medicaid spending increases, but it will not be possible to ascertain the motives leading to other changes in payment updates or methods.

A second cause of rising Medicaid expenditures, which from spending data alone cannot be easily distinguished from payment increases, is the recent spread of "provider donations" and "provider-specific taxes." Although the use of provider donations can be traced back to West Virginia in 1986, widespread adoption of these techniques came more recently after the law was clarified in the courts and Congress prohibited the Secretary of Health and Human Services (HHS) from directly regulating them (2).

The following illustration captures the spirit of these innovative financing programs. Hospitals, for example, may either donate funds to the state or pay a special state tax levied on hospitals. The revenue from this source is then earmarked for the Medicaid program by the state. Simultaneously, the state declares an increase in hospital reimbursement, which as new spending qualifies for additional federal matching payments. The federal payment could range from one to four times the size of the initial transaction, depending on the state-specific matching rate. As long as the increase in hospital reimbursement is equal to their donations or taxes, the hospitals are no worse off, as a group. Similarly, from the state's perspective, the donations or taxes financed the reimbursement increase without the use of additional state funds. The federal funds, however, represent a gain that can be shared in any proportion between the state and the hospitals. In some states, there has been a direct relationship between the donations or taxes of particular providers and the returns in reimbursement from the state. In others, there has been no such relationship.

According to a survey by the American Public Welfare Association, in 1991, 16 states had programs that would generate roughly $2.3 billion in additional federal matching funds, for a total of $4 billion in Medicaid financing (see Table 2). Some of this total supported increases in provider reimbursement that were in addition to payments that would have been made otherwise. Another portion supported eligibility expansions, a form of added spending discussed previously. The survey also inquired about the states' plans for fiscal year 1992. Table 3 summarizes the plans of 28 states whose programs would raise about $6 billion in additional federal matching funds for a total of nearly $10 billion in Medicaid spending. The escalation for 1992 suggests that there is good reason to expect additional costs per beneficiary as a cause of Medicaid spending growth over and above enrollment increases.

Congress recently attempted to limit the extent of these practices in the Medicaid Voluntary Contribution and Provider Specific Tax Amendments of 1991, which took effect on January 1, 1992. The law allowed the Secretary to deny federal matching for cases where there is a clear link between provider contributions and subsequent payments. It also capped the relative contribution these methods could make to qualifying "state share" subject to federal matching funds. Because not all the methods have such a direct linkage, and because the regulations are so recent, the future course of the provider donations and taxes issue is highly uncertain.

CONCLUSION

By any reasonable standard of comparison, Medicaid spending has indeed been soaring in recent years, to as much as a 26 percent increase for 1991. Part of the explanation is that Medicaid, the same as any other third-party payer for health care services, faces the pressures of rising health care prices, increased utilization, and costlier technologies. When the contributions of these factors and the modest trend of enrollment growth established between 1980 and 1988 are accounted for, one can explain about 10 to 11 percentage points of any recent year's overall growth rate.

Over and above this baseline, most of the additional spending growth for both 1990 and 1991 is explained by the fact that the program served substantially more people in each year—over 1.5 million (or 7.5 percent) more in 1990 and an additional 3.0 million (or 12 percent) in 1991. Part of this expansion is accounted for by the federally mandated eligibility expansions for pregnant women and children. Another part is due to expanding participation in public assistance programs, including Medicaid. It is not yet clear whether this expansion is a temporary one driven by the recession, or whether it is a structural shift. One possible cause of some added participation may be the public education and eligibility outreach programs undertaken by the states.

A final source of additional spending, although of limited impact through 1991, is the increases in provider payments, especially to hospitals.

It is difficult to identify which of these might have taken place anyway, which were induced by the Boren Amendment, and which were undertaken solely because they could be financed under provider tax and donation programs. In 1991, the additional spending from this source might have been $2 billion to $4 billion, or roughly 3 to 5 percentage points of the 26 percent overall growth in Medicaid spending. However, this activity expanded substantially in 1992 and surely accounts for a significant share of the even greater spending increase predicted for this year.

APPENDIX

Data

The principal data source for this chapter is the Health Care Financing Administration (HCFA) Form 2082 statistics collected from the state Medicaid programs annually by the HCFA. These data, available from 1975 through 1991, provide Medicaid expenditures and recipients by type of service (for example, inpatient hospital) and by reason of eligibility (for example, AFDC adult receiving cash assistance). In addition to totals for the entire program, detail is provided for every state or other jurisdiction. The Form 2082 data provide all of the counts of Medicaid beneficiaries that are used here, as well as the 1980–1988 baseline series of spending data (Figure 5, the underlying calculations for decomposition in Figure 6, and Table 1).

In contrast, the figures on total program spending and its percentage growth rates since 1988 (Figures 1, 2, 3, 4, and 6) are from the HCFA Form 64 data and related budget statistics and actuarial projections based on reports of state expenditures subject to federal matching funds. Although this latter source is viewed as the more reliable for expenditures, it does not provide information on beneficiaries and their characteristics. Therefore, Medicaid research often involves "mixing and matching" from these (not altogether consistent or compatible) data sources.

Until recently, the Form 2082 and the Form 64 data provided reasonably similar figures for total Medicaid spending, aside from well-understood differences in definition. Specifically, the Form 2082 data are based solely on tabulations of claims, or "medical vendor payments," while in addition to claims, the Form 64 data include premiums to Medicare and managed care organizations, lump sum adjustments handled outside the claims payment systems, and administrative costs. In recent years, Form 2082 totals were 10 to 11 percent below program totals from the Form 64 (see Table A.1.). Almost one half of this difference was due to administrative costs of around 5 percent (not shown). In 1991, however, Form 2082 spending was 17 percent, or $15 billion, below the program total.

Although a thorough investigation of this abruptly wider difference is beyond the scope of this paper, a quick look provides a suggestion of one source of higher Medicaid spending growth. Using the past two years' rate of 11.1 percent expected difference between the Form 64 data and the Form 2082 data, the discrepancy would have been expected to be about $10.2 billion ($91.9 billion times .111) in 1991. Therefore, the unexpected spending accounted for by the Form 64s, but not measured in the Form 2082s, is about $5 billion ($15.2 billion total difference less the $10.2 billion expected difference).

Table A.1. Comparison of total Medicaid spending from alternative sources, 1988–1991.

Year	Total Medicaid Spending (in billions)		Difference Between Form 64 and Form 2082	
	Form 64	Form 2082	Absolute (in millions)	Percent of 64
1988	54.1	48.7	5.4	9.9
1989	61.3	54.5	6.8	11.1
1990	72.9	64.9	8.1	11.1
1991	91.9	76.7	15.2	16.5

Source: HCFA Form 64, as adjusted for budget reports, and Form 2082.

Comparing discrepancies by service type between the two sources, inpatient hospital services (which in 1990 were reported with less than a $1 billion difference) differ by about the same $5 billion (the total difference for 1991 is about $6 billion, or $5 billion more than the previous year). Part or all of this could be explained by disproportionate share payments to hospitals, financed by Medicaid provider taxes and donations, many of which would have been paid as lump sums to hospitals, rather than in the form of rate adjustments. The lump sum payments would show up in the Form 64, but not in the Form 2082 claims-based system. On the other hand, some of the disproportionate share payments may have served as substitutes for rate increases that would have been granted otherwise. Therefore, the $5 billion is an upper-bound estimate of increased cost per beneficiary in excess of "baseline" spending growth.

Methods

In order to decompose the overall growth of Medicaid spending into its various causes, a simple econometric model of total spending was estimated. The coefficients of the model were then used to "predict" how spending would have grown in recent years under alternative assumptions—for example, about the increased number of beneficiaries. In this way, the influence of a particular cause can be identified, while the effects of others are held constant.

Calculations such as these can be very sensitive to the exact specification of the model and the assumptions made. Moreover, with only two or three annual data points of departure from the trend, it is difficult even to distinguish a real change from an apparent one due to a one-year anomaly in the data. Therefore, the decomposition shown in Figure 6 should be thought of as a "rough estimate," not an exact calculation. The data better support the qualitative statements made than they do the quantitative point estimates chosen.

The Econometric Model

With all of the detail available from the Form 2082 data, there is an overwhelming amount of choice among ways of modeling Medicaid spending over time. The topic of the current analysis limits the choices substantially, however. To be useful for prediction, the model may only contain independent variables whose future values can be known or predicted. An extremely simple approach was chosen—specifically, to model total program spending as a function of total people served by the program (beneficiaries) and the level of prices. This latter variable was chosen to measure the combined influence of prices and utilization, as discussed in the text. Various functional forms were estimated, along with two measures of cost per beneficiary—that is, the Consumer Price Index (CPI) and the Medical Care component of the Consumer Price Index (MCCPI). Finally, various time periods were considered. Because the late 1970s were still a period of rapid transfer of state-only funded activities to Medicaid, these years were omitted. The period 1980 to 1988 was chosen for the baseline estimates as most likely to represent the forces shaping the Medicaid program had the recent eligibility, reimbursement, and financing changes not taken place.

The estimated equation selected is shown in Table A.2. It is linear in the natural logarithm (log) of spending which is regressed on the log of beneficiaries and the MCCPI. When estimated in this form, the interpretation of any coefficient is that of an elasticity. For example, for each one percent change in annual beneficiaries, there will be a 1.024 percent change in spending (see Table A.2). Because this coefficient is so close to 1.00, the marginal beneficiary costs approximately the same as the average beneficiary. Foreshadowing this relationship are the proportions of beneficiary growth between

Table A.2. Regression for natural logarithm of total Medicaid spending, 1980–1988.

Variable	Estimate	t-statistic
Intercept	1.988	0.47
Log Recipients	1.024	3.95
Log MCCPI	1.065	30.22
R-Square = 0.997		

Source: Author's estimates using HCFA Form 2082 data.

1980 and 1988 cited in the text—specifically, 20 percent net disabled (after accounting for the decline in the elderly and recognizing their similar average costs) and 80 percent AFDC adults and children. If the marginal beneficiaries within each eligibility group had spending similar to that of the average ones, the 1:4 proportions were similar to those of the program as a whole, implying a marginal cost per beneficiary about equal to the average cost per beneficiary.

The preferred variable as a measure of the combined effects of prices and utilization on spending is the MCCPI. Judging from the estimated coefficient, which is also close to 1.00, increases in Medicaid payment to providers taken alone must have fallen below general increases in medical prices (as measured by the index), provided that there were also increases in utilization or "intensity" of service in Medicaid (as measured in other health insurance programs).

The Decomposition

The calculations underlying Figure 6, which divide the aggregate percent increases in Medicaid spending from official budget statistics into four categories, are based largely on the above estimates and Form 2082 beneficiary data. Specifically, the total change is divided into the following sources, in this order:

- The increase in spending that would have taken place if the 1980–1988 rate of increase and mix of beneficiaries had persisted, all other factors held at their previous year's levels.

- The increase in spending that would have taken place if the MCCPI had increased by its observed amount for the year, all other factors held at their previous year's levels. The sum of these first two effects is termed the "trend effect."

- The increase in spending that would have resulted from the excess of the observed beneficiary growth for the year over the historical rate, as predicted by the modeled relationship, all other factors held at their previous year's levels.

- The remaining increase (residual) is attributed to other causes.

The first of these listed effects explains just under one percentage point of the overall growth each year. It is the product of the historical growth rate in enrollment of 0.8 percent and the recipiency elasticity that is close to 1.0. The second and third effects are illustrated in Table A.3, which shows the actual and the predicted values for 1988 through 1991 that were plotted in Figure 5. To facilitate the translation between the lower Form 2082 spending base and the higher Form 64 spending levels, the percent increases in the predicted values from year to year were calculated (see Table A.3). The second effect for each year is the percent increase from the "enrollment trend" predictions, minus the first effect. The third effect for each year is the difference between the percent increase for the "actual enrollment" predictions and the percent increase for the "enrollment trend" predictions. The fourth effect was calculated as a residual. Its absolute value in spending was also judged "reasonable" when compared to the American Public Welfare Association survey data on 1991 taxes and donations and to the Form 64/Form 2082 discrepancy calculations discussed above.

Table A. 3. Actual and predicted Medicaid spending under alternative assumptions.

| Year | Actual | | Predicted[a] | | | |
| | | | 1980–1988 Enrollment Trends[b] | | Actual Enrollment[c] | |
	Spending (in billions)	Percent Increase	Spending (in billions)	Percent Increase	Spending (in billions)	Percent Increase
1988	48.7	—	48.2	—	48.2	—
1989	54.5	11.9	52.4	8.7	53.6	11.2
1990	64.9	19.0	57.9	10.6	63.2	18.0
1991	76.7	18.2	63.8	10.2	77.5	22.7

Source: Author's estimates using HCFA Form 2082 data.

Notes: a. Total spending for medical vendor payments from 2082 data.
b. Based on regression estimates in Table A-2. Assumes 1980–88 enrollment trend persists through 1991 and uses actual increases in MCCPI for each year.
c. Based on regression estimates in Table A-2. Assumes actual enrollment and actual increases in MCCPI for each year.

ADDITIONAL READING

American Public Welfare Association. *Medicaid Funding Programs That Tax Medical Providers* (Washington, D.C.: Medicaid Management Institute, American Public Welfare Association, September 26, 1991).

American Public Welfare Association. *Voluntary Contributions and Provider-Specific Taxes—Survey Results* (Washington, D.C.: Medicaid Management Institute, American Public Welfare Association, August 26, 1991).

Levit, K.R., et al. "National Health Expenditures, 1990." *Health Care Financing Review* 13,1 (Fall 1991), pp. 29–54.

Sonnefeld, S.T., et al. "Projections of National Health Expenditures through the Year 2000." *Health Care Financing Review* 13, 1 (Fall 1991), pp. 1–27.

U.S. Department of Labor, Bureau of Labor Statistics. *Monthly Labor Review,* various issues.

U.S. House of Representatives, Committee on Ways and Means. *1992 Green Book: Background Materials and Data on Programs Within the Jurisdiction of the Committee on Ways and Means* (Washington, D.C.: U.S. Government Printing Office, WMCP:102–44, May 15, 1992).

REFERENCES

1. Prospective Payment Assessment Commission. *Medicaid Hospital Payment: Congressional Report* (Washington, D.C.: Prospective Payment Assessment Commission, C-91-02, October 1, 1991).

2. Merlis, M. *Medicaid: Provider Donations and Provider-Specific Taxes* (Washington, D.C.: Congressional Research Service, 91–722 EPW, October 2, 1991).

•

2

Understanding the Recent Growth in Medicaid Spending

JOHN HOLAHAN,
TERESA COUGHLIN, LEIGHTON KU,
DAVID HESLAM,
COLIN WINTERBOTTOM

INTRODUCTION

This chapter examines Medicaid spending growth over the last six or seven years and suggests a number of explanations for that growth. The information reported is based on interviews conducted with over 100 officials in nine states from April to June 1992. The interviews included state Medicaid directors, budget officials, state legislators, and representatives of provider and advocacy groups to gain a variety of perspectives. The following represents the authors' interpretation of the major changes that have occurred in Medicaid over the past several years.

By any standard, Medicaid costs have exploded since 1988, causing considerable alarm at federal and state levels. This rapid growth was in contrast to experience in earlier years. Medicaid spending between 1980 and 1988 had increased more slowly than the increase in national personal health care expenditures (9.7 percent versus 10.4 percent annually), despite serving a population of low-income families and chronically ill, disabled, and elderly individuals (1). Moreover, Medicaid spending on acute care services grew significantly more slowly than national acute care spending and only slightly in excess of the rate of inflation.

In 1989, however, Medicaid spending jumped by 11.9 percent in comparison with national spending increases of 10.6 percent. Medicaid spending increased by another 19.9 percent in 1990, by 30.1 percent in 1991, 30 percent in 1992 (2) reaching $114 billion. Why were states so successful in containing costs prior to 1989? And what has happened to change the course of Medicaid spending in the last three years? Some observers have suggested that the recent cost explosion is due to the large number of federal mandates that were passed beginning in the mid-1980s, but we suggest that Medicaid spending is very complex and that there are many other important factors that have contributed to the recent expenditure surge. Furthermore, we found that there is no single set of factors that explain the growth in Medicaid in every state.

Before turning to the reasons for this growth, we present a few tables that illustrate where this growth has occurred. Table 1 shows enrollment and spending growth by broad eligibility categories (3). The data are divided into two periods: 1984 to 1987 and 1987 to 1991. Medicaid spending clearly began to accelerate after 1987. What is different about the latter period is that spending growth on adults and children was faster than for the aged and blind and disabled. While a much larger amount of money was spent on the aged and blind and disabled, for the first time in recent history, the rates of increase in spending on adults and children were greater.

Table 2 indicates one reason for this trend: enrollment growth of adults and children grew at 6.0 and 6.6 percent annually, respectively. These growth rates are consistent with the expected effects of the federally mandated expansion of Medicaid coverage for pregnant women and children. However, as is shown in Table 3, while the rate of spending increase has been higher for adults and children in recent years, spending on the disabled and aged account for most, nearly two thirds, of the recent increases in actual dollars spent by the Medicaid program.

Table 1. National Medicaid expenditures by eligibility group.

Eligibility Group	Expend. in 1984 (in billions)	Annual % Growth 1984–87	Annual % Growth 1987–91	Expend. in 1991 (in billions)
All	**$35.5**	**9.5%**	**16.9%**	**$87.1**
Adults	4.5	6.5	20.7	11.5
Aged	12.7	8.3	14.0	27.3
Bl & Dis	11.9	11.7	16.7	30.9
Children	4.4	10.6	22.1	13.2

Table 2. National Medicaid enrollees by eligibility group.

Eligibility Group	Enrollees in 1984 (in millions)	Annual % Growth 1984–87	Annual % Growth 1987–91	Enrollees in 1991 (in millions)
All	**24.1**	**1.9%**	**5.6%**	**31.7**
Adults	5.6	1.4	6.0	7.3
Aged	3.3	0.2	1.7	3.5
Bl & Dis	3.1	4.7	4.9	4.3
Children	12.1	1.8	6.6	16.5

Table 3. National Medicaid expenditures per enrollee by eligibility group.

Eligibility Group	Expend. per Enr. in 1984	Annual % Growth 1984–87	Annual % Growth 1987–91	Expend. per Enr. in 1991
All	**$1,473**	**5.6%**	**10.7%**	**$2,748**
Adults	803	3.8	13.9	1,567
Aged	3,884	6.0	12.1	7,745
Bl & Dis	3,882	5.0	11.3	7,121
Children	363	6.4	14.5	799

Table 4. National Medicaid expenditures by type of service.

Type of Service	Expenditures in 1991 (in billions)	Annual Percent Change 1987–1991
All Services	**$87.1**	**16.9%**
Inpatient Hospital Services	25.6	22.5
Nursing Facility Services	20.8	11.4
Physicians' Services/ Laboratory & Radiology	5.4	13.7
Outpatient Hospital Services	6.1	20.2
Intermediate Care Facility (MR)	8.2	10.4
Mental Health Facility Services	2.3	17.3
Home Health Services	4.7	23.1
Prescription Drugs	5.7	16.7
Medicare Payments	2.0	27.6
HMO & Group Health Payments	1.9	20.1
Other Services	4.4	21.4

Table 4 shows spending growth by service type. Here it can be seen that spending increases were broadly spread across many different types of services. Hospital inpatient and outpatient spending (particularly on adults and children) grew at rates well above increases in inflation, which was about 6 percent during the 1987 to 1991 period. (As we will discuss below, spending growth for some services, particularly hospitals, may be distorted because of provider tax and donation and disproportionate share programs.) Spending on prescription drugs and home health services also increased markedly, growing by 16.7 and 23.1 percent, respectively. Payments to health maintenance organizations (HMOs) and other prepaid health plans increased by 20.1 percent per year as states attempted to increase the use of managed care. Payments to Medicare also increased sharply (27.6 percent), reflecting increased payments of premiums and cost sharing for poor elderly. The 18.2 percent annual increase in other spending reflects increases in dental care, medical supplies, other practitioners, and other services. In sum, growth rates for most services were well in excess of annual growth rates in enrollment and inflation.

Table 5 shows the growth in spending by state. The states are organized by geographic area to highlight regional differences in growth rates. New England states, for example, have the fastest growth rates, probably reflecting the severe effects of the recession in this region. Similarly, southern states showed high growth rates. Most likely this reflects the fact that southern states historically have had restrictive eligibility standards. They have been, therefore, more affected by the federal mandates of the mid-1980s, which increased program enrollment and consequently have had faster growth rates in both enrollment and spending. The remaining states have generally had slower growth rates either because they have had broad eligibility standards for many years and thus had not been affected as much by the federal mandates or because they had not been seriously affected by the recession by 1991.

Table 5. Recent Medicaid enrollment and expenditure trends by region: average annual growth rates, 1987–1991.

Region	Enrollment	Expenditures Per Enrollee	Total Expenditures
New England	4.4%	18.2%	23.4%
Middle Atlantic	2.3	12.2	14.8
South Atlantic	10.4	10.2	21.7
East South Central	7.4	13.8	22.2
West South Central	11.1	8.2	20.3
East North Central	3.7	8.6	12.6
West North Central	5.6	10.4	16.5
Mountain	9.5	6.7	16.8
Pacific	3.4	10.2	13.9
U.S. Total	5.6	10.7	16.9

Site Visits

To explore the reasons for the recent growth in Medicaid, the authors conducted a set of site visits to nine states: California, Connecticut, Florida, Maryland, Michigan, Missouri, New York, South Carolina, and Texas. These states were selected on the basis of five criteria. The interest was in states that, first, accounted for a large share of national Medicaid expenditures; second, that historically had used very different approaches to establishing eligibility standards enabling assessment of the impacts of mandates to cover pregnant women and children and the elderly; third, that had been affected in varying degrees by the current economic recession; fourth, that had adopted different approaches to provider donations and tax programs; and fifth, that were geographically diverse. The key characteristics of the study states are summarized in Table 6.

Table 6. Select characteristics of states in which site visits were conducted.

State	Region	Program Generosity (1986)	Impact of Mandates and Options[2]	Response to Mandates and Options[3]	Fiscal Capacity (1986)[4]	Percent change in Unemployment (1987–1991)	Expected Reliance on Provider Donations and Tax Programs
California	Far West	High	Low	High	High	Small Increase (4%)	Low
Connecticut	Northeast	High	Low	High	High	Large Increase (103%)	Moderate
Florida	Southeast	Low-Moderate	Moderate	Moderate-High	Moderate-High	Large Increase (22%)	Moderate
Maryland	Mideast	Moderate	Moderate	High	Moderate-High	Large Increase (28%)	Moderate-High
Michigan	Midwest	Moderate	Low	Moderate-High	Moderate	Small Increase (12%)	High
Missouri	Plains	Low	High	Low	Moderate	Small Increase (5%)	High
New York	Mideast	High	Low	Moderate-High	Moderate	Large Increase (47%)	Low
South Carolina	Southeast	Moderate-Low	Moderate	High	Low	Large Decrease (-31%)	High
Texas	Southwest	Low-Moderate	High	Low	Moderate-High	Small Decrease (-6%)	Moderate-High

1. Program generosity was judged using a combination of three criteria: a) payment per Medicaid recipient 1986; b) AFDC eligibility threshold as a percent of poverty, 1987; and c) presence and generosity of medically needy program, 1986.

2. Impact of OBRA 1986, 1987, 1989, and MCCA 1988 pregnant women and children mandates and options was judged by how far the state had to expand to meet the mandates' provisions.

3. Response to mandates and options was judged by: a) how rapidly the state adopted options; and b) to what extent they adopted options.

4. Fiscal capacity was judged using four criteria: a) 1986 per capita personal income; b) percent population below poverty line in 1986; c) state and local tax capacity; and d) state and local tax effort.

REASONS FOR MEDICAID SPENDING GROWTH

This investigation indicates several reasons for Medicaid spending growth in recent years. These include the federal mandates covering pregnant women and children, as well as new legislative mandates, the recession, rising health care costs, the aging of the population, and state efforts to shift previously state-funded services into Medicaid. A major factor permitting states to finance the recent surge in Medicaid spending has been provider tax and donation programs and the related use of disproportionate share payments to providers, primarily hospitals. These initiatives have not only enabled states to expand Medicaid coverage and benefits without large tax increases, but have also enabled states to help hospitals provide uncompensated care.

The Federal Mandates: Pregnant Women and Children

Since the mid-1980s, Congress has enacted a broad array of initiatives mandating states to expand both Medicaid program eligibility and benefits. Many believe that these mandates have been the single largest contributor to the growth in Medicaid spending that has occurred since 1987. Virtually each year's Budget Reconciliation Act, beginning with the Deficit Reduction Act (DEFRA) legislation in 1984, included new Medicaid expansions. Many of these expansions were targeted to pregnant women and children. Starting in 1985, for example, Medicaid programs were required to cover first-time pregnant women and infants who met Medicaid financial eligibility standards and to phase in coverage of children meeting Aid to Families with Dependent Children (AFDC) income standards up to age five, regardless of family structure. The Omnibus Budget Reconciliation Act of 1986 (1986 OBRA) legislation permitted states to cover pregnant women and infants up to age one in families at 100 percent of the poverty level or less. It permitted states the option of expanding Medicaid coverage up to age five in families with income less than 100 percent of poverty. The 1986 legislation also provided states with the option of covering elderly and disabled individuals up to 100 percent of poverty.

The 1987 OBRA legislation went further by permitting states to cover pregnancy-related services for individuals up to 185 percent of poverty as well as infants up to age one. Then in 1988, the Medicare Catastrophic Act required mandatory coverage of pregnant women and infants under age one up to 100 percent of poverty. This new coverage was to be phased in over time, with full coverage by July 1, 1990. The 1989 OBRA legislation required expansion of coverage of pregnant women, infants, and children up to age six in families with income up to 133 percent of the poverty line. The 1990 OBRA legislation required phasing in coverage of children through age 18 whose families have income up to 100 percent of poverty. The age limit now set at eight will increase annually by one year over the next 10 years.

Among our study states, all indicated that the mandates to cover pregnant women and children had important effects on enrollment and expenditures. This was particularly true, as we expected, in Florida, South Carolina, and Texas. But the other states also indicated that these mandates had significant effects on their programs. It was clear, however, that assessing the true impacts of the mandates was difficult because most of the mandated changes were being implemented at the same time that the recession was also causing an increase in enrollment. For example, state officials in Connecticut, New York, Maryland, and Missouri believed that the recession contributed more to program expenditure growth than did the pregnant women and children mandates, though in reality it is difficult to disentangle the effect of each.

In an effort to try to measure the individual effects of the mandates and the recession, we conducted simulations using the Urban Institute's TRIM2 microsimulation model. The microsimulation model allowed us to ask the question: What would Medicaid enrollment and expenditures have been if the mandates had never been enacted? We used the model to impose the 1985 eligibility rules on the 1990 population and economy, focusing on the changes for pregnant women and children. That is, the simulation allowed us to control for the higher unemployment rates and increased numbers of people in poverty, because the 1985 eligibility rules were imposed on the population in 1990. We also controlled for inflation and changes in benefits because 1990 Medicaid costs per enrollee are used.

The results for this simulation are shown in Table 7. They demonstrate that Medicaid enrollment of nonelderly Americans increased by 13.2 percent relative to enrollment levels that would have existed had the mandates not been imposed. We estimate that spending on acute care services for the nonelderly would have increased by $3.8 billion, or by 11.2 percent, because of the added enrollment. Table 7 also shows that the increases in enrollment and cost were greatest in the south, midwest, and mountain states, whereas growth was slowest in the northeast and far west, reflecting historical patterns of the breadth of Medicaid coverage. Thus, since total Medicaid spending increased from $39.1 billion to $68.9 billion between 1985 and 1990, the simulation results suggest that the increase due to the mandates accounted for only 12.8 percent of the growth. Even after adjusting for increases in national medical care price inflation, the mandates still account for only about 22 percent of the growth in Medicaid spending. This estimate actually overstates the effects of the mandates, because many states, on their own initiative, were already covering these newly entitled populations. Clearly, there are a number of other factors that are important in explaining recent Medicaid expenditure increases.

Other Federal Mandates

In addition to the pregnant women and children mandates, other federally legislated expansions were passed in the mid-to-late-1980s. These other

Table 7. Simulation of Medicaid enrollment and costs under alternative eligibility rules: 1990 nonelderly population; 1985 and 1990 eligibility rules (persons in thousands, dollars in millions).

Region	1985 Eligibility Rules		1990 Eligibility Rules		Percentage Increase In:	
	Average Monthly Enrollment	Annual Expenditures	Average Monthly Enrollment	Annual Expenditures	Average Monthly Enrollment	Annual Expenditures
New England	886	$1,721.6	944	$1,830.3	6.5%	6.3%
Middle Atlantic	3,123	7,738.8	3,427	8,272.6	9.7	6.9
East North Central	3,250	4,906.1	3,745	5,832.9	15.2	18.9
West North Central	967	1,675.2	1,209	1,899.2	25.1	13.4
South Atlantic	2,792	5,024.9	3,283	5,891.7	17.6	17.3
East South Central	1,331	3,413.5	1,598	3,786.5	20.	10.9
West South Central	2,032	3,229.4	2,285	3,422.1	12.5	6.0
Mountain	459	679.4	578	825.5	26.1	21.5
Pacific	3,930	5,359.8	4,169	5,780.6	6.1	7.8
U.S. Total	18,770	$33,748.6	21,239	$37,541.3	13.2%	11.2%

mandates, affecting the elderly and the disabled, also potentially contributed to the growth in expenditures. The Medicare Catastrophic Coverage Act (MCCA), for example, required that states pay the premiums and cost-sharing for Medicare beneficiaries with incomes under 100 percent of poverty. This requirement was to be phased in and fully implemented by January 1, 1992. More recently, states have been required to accelerate these provisions and to pay cost sharing for the elderly between 100 percent and 120 percent of poverty. The MCCA also required states to protect a minimum level of assets and income of individuals remaining in the community when a spouse enters a nursing home. The 1989 OBRA legislation expanded the Early and Periodic Screening, Diagnosis, and Treatment Programs (EPSDT) for children by requiring states to pay for a wide range of services, even if their Medicaid plan does not cover the service, if a qualified provider says the service is medically necessary. The 1987 OBRA legislation had enacted a number of provisions requiring states to improve the quality of nursing home care and to assure that reimbursement rates would reflect the increased costs of the necessary improvements. These provisions are being phased in and should be fully reflected in Medicaid spending in 1992.

In addition to these mandates, the federal government in the late 1980s also expanded Medicaid coverage to entirely new populations: newly legalized aliens and undocumented persons who otherwise would not have been entitled to Medicaid. These expansions were mandated in the 1986 Immigration Reform and Control Act (IRCA) and 1986 OBRA legislation, respectively.

These additional mandates were not generally believed to be as important as those affecting pregnant women and children. The expanded coverage of the elderly, for example, has been important in some states but not in others, principally because many states have not actively implemented this legislation. The effects of the EPSDT provisions are only beginning to be felt, though state officials maintained that the EPSDT will need to be greatly expanded. Despite this expected expansion, the EPSDT benefit constitutes a relatively small part of the program; thus, this mandate should not have a large effect on total Medicaid spending.

The nursing home reform provisions should increase Medicaid spending in some states, but many states had already adopted these reform provisions on their own. The spousal impoverishment provisions of MCCA were believed to be potentially important, but at this time there is no real evidence of their fiscal impact. Anecdotal evidence, however, is now mounting that some non-poor elderly are using estate planning techniques to shelter assets and qualify for Medicaid without first "spending down" to poverty. State officials in Connecticut, New York, California, and Florida all acknowledge that this was a problem, but they did not know the magnitude.

Other provisions in 1990 OBRA legislation affecting full-cost reimbursement for federally qualified health centers have raised per visit costs substantially, but these increased costs are not significant in terms of total spending. The 1986 OBRA legislation requiring coverage of undocumented persons and the IRCA mandate covering newly legalized aliens seem to have been important only in California. These provisions alone reportedly accounted for 350,000 new enrollees in MediCal at an estimated cost of $1 billion in 1992. In sum, while these other mandates have contributed to the growth in Medicaid spending, we believe that the mandates with the most important national impact during this period are those affecting pregnant women and children.

Rising Health Care Costs

In addition to the federal mandates, the states also have been affected by the rapid rise in health care costs that is occurring nationally. For example, between 1988 and 1989, national health spending for personal health care services increased about 10.6 percent (4). About 6.7 percent of the growth in spending nationally was due to the increase in health care prices; most of the remainder, about 4 percent per year, was due to increases in utilization. This is consistent across hospital, physician, dental, and other services. Home health care is an exception, with utilization increasing substantially faster than increases in price.

Medicaid programs in the past have generally not kept up with the increase in health care prices, but there is increasing pressure on the states to do so. With payment rates to hospitals, physicians, and other providers well below market rates, states risk further deteriorations in access if rates do not keep up with the growth in private charges. That is, Medicaid rates do not have to increase to the levels of private charges, but failure to increase at the same rates risks further reductions in access to providers.

Moreover, the states are under increasing legal pressure to raise payment rates. In a number of states, e.g., California, Connecticut, Michigan, Missouri, New York, and Texas, hospitals and/or nursing homes have been successful in bringing suits to increase state payment rates in line with provisions of the Boren Amendment, which states that Medicaid providers be paid rates sufficient to cover the costs of efficiently and economically operated facilities. Even states that have not been sued, such as Florida, Maryland, and South Carolina, have been affected because of the fear of Boren Amendment challenges in their own states. Medical societies and welfare rights organizations have also been successful in bringing suits against Medicaid programs, e.g., California, to increase fees paid to physicians, dentists, and other providers.

Prescription drugs present special problems for Medicaid programs. Prescription drugs have been one of the fastest rising expenditure categories in the Medicaid program throughout the 1980s. The 1990 OBRA legislation required drug manufacturers to provide rebates to the states comparable to the discounts provided to other large, high-volume purchasers. The legislation, however, also imposed a number of requirements on the states. Among other things, it required the states to cover most new drugs for six months, restricted use of formularies, placed limits on payment reductions, and imposed requirements to implement education programs for pharmacies and prescribers on drug interactions. The states' savings because of the drug rebate program has been mixed. Most believe they have received some savings from the rebates. They also believe, however, that drug manufacturers have increased their prices to other large, high-volume purchasers to which the rebates are tied. In addition, they believe the restrictions imposed by the legislation have limited their ability to control utilization and have added greatly to their administrative burdens. Other evidence is similarly discouraging. The Congressional Research Service estimates that drug expenditures increased by 21 percent in 1991, after rebates, which is higher than any year from 1987 to 1990 (5).

Medicaid Maximization

Some of the growth in Medicaid spending has been "intentional." The states have found Medicaid's matching funds an attractive source of revenue for financing services that previously had been part of state-only funded programs. For example, the expansion of institutional care for the mentally retarded in the early 1980s reflected policies to substitute Medicaid funds for care historically provided by the state. Expansion of home- and community-based care in Medicaid has substituted in part for personal care services that traditionally had been funded through the Title XX program. Likewise, expansion of coverage of pregnant women, as required by the new federal mandates, is in part replacing state spending on maternal and child health programs, or is permitting these funds to be used for other purposes such as case management or outreach programs. In a few states, the deinstitutionalization of the mentally ill resulted in a shift of individuals between the ages of 21 and 64 out of state-run institutions, where they were not eligible for Medicaid, into the community, where they are eligible for the Supplementary Security Income (SSI) program and, thus, federal income support, as well as for Medicaid acute care benefits. In these cases, increases in Medicaid spending offset spending that the states would have otherwise made.

Although the incentives to shift state-only expenses to Medicaid have long existed, it was our impression that the states were rapidly learning how to include various services in Medicaid in the late 1980s and early 1990s. Part of the reason may have been the increasing fiscal pressure of state deficits and increasing sophisticated knowledge about Medicaid rules and regulations. Even so, there were substantial differences in the extent to which the states had attempted to redefine services to fit under the Medicaid umbrella. New York has been very assertive in this direction, while Texas and California have been, heretofore, less aggressive.

The Aged and Chronically Ill

Yet another factor contributing to Medicaid spending increases is the increased demand for services among the aged and chronically ill. This has resulted in growing pressure to expand long-term care services in virtually every state we visited. Many states also face similar pressures to expand services for the disabled. A major role of the Medicaid program historically has been to finance long-term institutional care for the elderly and chronically ill. In general, Medicaid expenditures for institutional long-term care services have slowed over the last few years as compared to prior years. This slowing reflects the fact that most mentally retarded children and adults (as well as many of the mentally ill) had been shifted from state institutions to Medicaid-funded facilities in previous years. This shift caused a big surge in spending in the mid-1980s. Now that the shift is virtually complete, the spending growth rate has leveled. In addition, the states have restricted, through direct regulation and payment policy, the growth in the supply of nursing home beds. More recently, efforts to move individuals out of institutions into the community may also be slowing the growth in spending for institutional care. Reflecting this deinstitutionalization trend, Medicaid spending for home health care and for home- and community-based waiver programs has expanded significantly, making spending for home health services the fastest growing benefit in Medicaid.

Other Factors Affecting Eligibility

Other forces besides the mandates and the recession have led to increased eligibility. Several states have streamlined eligibility processing by combining it with eligibility determination for other programs. This has allegedly increased program participation. Most states also began more extensive outstationing of Medicaid eligibility workers in hospitals and clinics. The states believed that not only did this increase enrollment, it also brought in higher-cost users, because the new enrollees were inherently service users, especially pregnant women. Next, recent legislation linking eligibility for many people to some percentage of the federal poverty level assures annual increases in the income standards. The states can no longer as readily affect eligibility by freezing or reducing AFDC payment standards. Finally, a recent Supreme Court decision affecting disabled children (Zebley *v.* Sullivan) has also increased enrollment of high-cost cases. Surprisingly, the states reported that while AIDS, drug abuse, homelessness, and other social problems have all contributed to the spending growth, they have contributed to a lesser extent than the other factors discussed earlier.

STATE RESPONSES TO MEDICAID GROWTH

In the past two or three years, the increases in Medicaid costs have come into sharp conflict with declining revenues because of the recession. In all states, Medicaid has become one of the largest and fastest growing programs in their budgets. Since most states have balanced budget requirements, the growth in Medicaid expenditures has led to several types of responses: increases in state taxes; constraints on other sectors of the budget; renewed Medicaid cost containment, including managed care; and enhancement of state revenues through use of Medicaid provider tax and donation programs.

Most states that were visited for this study had used a combination of these approaches, though the relative importance of each approach varied from state to state. All of these approaches are discussed here, but more emphasis is given to the last approach—disproportionate share programs—which have been a major factor in financing recent Medicaid growth.

State Tax Increases

Several states, e.g., California, Connecticut, Texas, and Maryland, have had to increase state taxes, such as income, sales, or property taxes, to help pay for Medicaid growth. Florida has been considering a tax increase. In some cases, county taxes are also affected. For example, in New York, where counties are responsible for about half of the non-federal cost of Medicaid, growth in Medicaid spending is considered a major cause of increases in county taxes. It is well known that tax increases are unpopular politically, so that the recent tax increases are a sign of the importance of Medicaid to the states and the difficulty that the states experience in reining in Medicaid costs. In some cases, the tax increases were required due to general state budget troubles, of which Medicaid was just one large component. In some other cases, tax increases were specifically linked to Medicaid or health care. For example, in California, a cigarette tax, among other things, went to fund the state-funded program that extends Medicaid coverage up to 200 percent of the federal poverty line.

Constraining Other Budget Sectors

Since Medicaid is an entitlement program that generates at least an equal level of federal matching dollars, the states are understandably reticent to cut Medicaid budgets. Other sectors of the budget, which are discretionary, such as higher education, or which are less popular, such as welfare, are more easily cut, both fiscally and politically. Table 8 reviews state budget trends for 1987–90. For the nation as well as for the states visited during this study, Medicaid was consistently a growing portion of the state budget, while other sectors, such as higher education, transportation, and cash assistance, tended to be shrinking as a proportion of the state budget.

Medicaid Cost Containment

In the past two years, state Medicaid officials have been designing and implementing new methods to contain costs. In most cases, these efforts

Table 8. State expenditures (including federal funds), all states by budget category.

Budget Category	State Expend. 1990 (in billions)	Annual Percentage Change 1987–1990	Change in Share of Total State Expend. 1987–1990
Elem. & Sec. Education	$115	7.5%	0.5%
Transportation	49	4.8	−6.9
Medicaid	62	13.9	19.4
Higher Education	61	7.1	−0.6
Total Cash Assistance	25	6.1	−3.5
Corrections	17	12.8	16.0
All Other	171	5.7	−4.5
Total Expenditures	**$501**	**7.3%**	N.A.

Source: National Association of State Budget Officers, *State Expenditure Report: 1989* (Washington, D.C.: NASBO, 1989); National Association of State Budget Officers, *State Expenditure Report: 1991* (Washington, D.C.: NASBO, 1991).

have not been in place prior to FY 1992, so that they are difficult to detect in historical financial data. There has been no single major retrenchment strategy. The states have generally implemented numerous small to moderate budget reductions, which add up to desired budget savings targets. Many of the states visited have adopted or are considering a variety of budget reduction approaches used during previous recessions, e.g., reductions in provider payments, restrictions on optional benefits, eligibility reductions, or efforts to reduce service utilization. However, unlike in previous economic downturns, the states now have less latitude in enacting cutbacks because of federal mandates that expanded eligibility, or pressures from court decisions that reduce the states' abilities to reduce institutional provider payment rates.

In most states, Medicaid eligibility has been relatively unaffected. Cutting optional eligibility is usually considered a last resort. Florida, for example, recently enacted a bill to completely eliminate its medically needy program, but this was reversed prior to implementation after a storm of vocal protests. On the other hand, the states have made serious reductions in cash assistance and medical benefits to their general relief populations, i.e., their state-only welfare and Medicaid programs. This group, largely made up of single men or childless couples, has little political clout and receives no federal matching dollars. However, Medicaid could still provide indirect assistance by helping to finance uncompensated care through disproportionate share programs.

A variety of incremental savings were achieved through targeted efforts to contain service costs. Although physician payment rates in Medicaid are generally quite low, they are still often a target for reductions, in part because they are less susceptible to Boren Amendment legal challenges.

Prescription drugs are the largest optional Medicaid benefit, but no states have seriously considered complete elimination of this benefit. Not only are drugs a popular benefit, but officials are concerned that complete elimination would not be cost-effective since patients without medications may end up in hospitals for more expensive care. Some states have tried to marginally reduce the costs of prescription drugs by adopting co-payments or limits on the number of prescriptions and so on. Certain smaller optional benefits, such as chiropractry or podiatry, are a target for reductions or elimination, but have limited savings potential. And, again, states realize that cutting these benefits may cause increased spending for physician services.

The final area that often arose in recent budget discussions is managed care. Several states are expanding the use of managed care, both in HMOs and Primary Care Case Management programs. However, with the exception of Michigan, there is little evidence of major savings because Medicaid acute care benefits and payment rates are not particularly high. Michigan believes it saves about 10 percent relative to fee-for-service expenses and intends to expand managed care to its entire Medicaid population over the next two years. New York projects a more modest 5 percent savings and plans to cover 50 percent of its caseload over the next several years. Other states have less ambitious plans for managed care expansion. State officials were more apt to believe that managed care was likely to improve the access and quality of care (and perhaps costs) by giving the recipients a usual source of care, as opposed to emergency rooms. Some states with significant rural populations are either uninterested in managed care (South Carolina) or plan to limit programs to large cities (Missouri).

Although the Medicaid budget is a large target for savings, the states find that it is difficult to make large reductions because of federal mandates, fear of court challenges, and the political or health policy appeal of the optional services. Finally, Medicaid budgets can only be cut to the extent that the states have optional services in the first place. Thus, some of the southern states which began with leaner Medicaid programs inherently have less potential to cut. For example, Texas had essentially no budget cuts in the past several years, despite several tax increases. Officials explained that this was, at least in part, because Texas did not have much to cut in the first place.

PROVIDER TAXES AND DONATIONS AND DISPROPORTIONATE SHARE PROGRAMS

Because of the large number of different pressures on Medicaid programs to expand enrollment and benefits, coupled with recent revenue pressures, the states have been increasingly creative in designing new methods of funding the program. Basically, the states have instituted new taxes on hospitals, or have required donations or contributions from hospitals, nursing homes, and other providers. In August of 1991, 29 states reported using donations and/or taxes to fund some part of their fiscal year

1992 Medicaid spending (5). The result is that the federal government now provides matching contributions to both provider donations or taxes, as well as to state general revenue contributions to the Medicaid program. These programs have eased state general fund contributions to the Medicaid program. At the same time, they have also helped the states to meet the federal mandates and to finance other program expansions both for historically covered eligibility groups and for the newly expanded groups. Provider donations and taxes have meant a large increase in federal dollars going to Medicaid, essentially similar in principle to an increase in the federal matching rate.

Provider tax and donation programs have been implemented in a variety of ways. The following example illustrates how provider donations and taxes have worked in some cases. Assume that a state has a certain reimbursement rate for a hospital—say $500 per day—and that the hospital provides Medicaid 1,000 days, resulting in $500,000 in Medicaid payments. Assuming a 50 percent matching rate, half would be paid by the state and the remainder by the federal government. Next, assume the state required a donation or imposed a tax on this hospital that would result in revenue of $200,000. The state would then raise its reimbursement rate to the hospital to $700 per day. The state then reports $700,000 in payments to this hospital, which results in a much larger federal match to the state ($350,000). The state then pays the hospital in part with federal funds ($350,000) and in part, in effect, by returning the donation or tax to the hospital ($200,000). The remainder, or $150,000, comes from the state's own funds. But the state now has a considerable amount of money ($100,000) left over that it had been paying to hospitals. It can use these funds to expand other Medicaid services, in which case it is eligible for additional federal matching payments, or to reduce taxes or to fund other services.

In many cases, disproportionate share programs have been critical to the "enhanced payment" component of these programs. By law, Medicaid hospital payments can not exceed Medicare levels, except for disproportionate share payments. Thus, if a state wants to pay much higher levels to targeted hospitals, it can use a disproportionate share program. These programs were originally intended to provide incremental assistance to hospitals, which provided disproportionate levels of care to low-income (i.e, Medicaid and uncompensated care) patients and which might, therefore, have more precarious financial status.

Disproportionate share payments to hospitals have thus been permitted and actually encouraged for several years, but the states have only recently become more aggressive and creative in using them. While there is a wide variety of approaches, the basic principles of how states are using these programs to their advantage are often similar. Essentially, a group of hospitals (or counties supporting the hospitals) makes a contribution to the state, which in turn makes disproportionate share payments to these and possibly other hospitals, obtaining federal matching payments in the process. These mechanisms have been used both to increase the overall payments to hospitals, thereby covering much of the uncompensated care provided by those hospitals, and to reduce a state's general fund deficits. In some states, these payments help states finance the hospital care for the same general assistance populations whose benefits they have recently reduced.

Provider tax and donation programs and disproportionate share programs are often linked, but need not be. Provider tax and donation programs are mechanisms to bring new, non- state-appropriated revenue into Medicaid, while disproportionate share programs are mechanisms to provide enhanced payments to a group of hospitals. Provider tax and donation programs can exist without disproportionate share and vice versa, although they are usually linked.

A few state examples will illustrate how these programs work. In 1991, Michigan hospitals made contributions of $401 million; the state in turn made disproportionate share payments to the same hospitals of $438 million. The state received approximately $240 million in federal matching contributions and had $203 million left over to pay for other services, or to reduce its general fund deficit. This disproportionate share payment contributed to a 34.9 percent increase in overall Medicaid payments at the same time that the state's own spending for Medicaid from its general funds declined by about 8 percent.

In 1991, Texas had four disproportionate share programs amounting to $1.2 billion. The largest was a program in which the 25 largest Medicaid-volume hospitals contribute 1.25 percent of their revenues to the state. The state received the federal match and allocated it in two portions. The bulk, 95 percent, was redirected to the 25 hospitals, which were predominantly public hospitals serving high volumes of poor patients. The remaining 5 percent of the funds was returned to 90 rural hospitals (the top 50 percent of rural hospitals with indigent care).

Beginning in May 1992, California established its Intergovernmental Transfer Payments program. Under the program, all counties with county hospitals (20 of the 58 counties have such hospitals), hospital districts, and selected University of California hospitals contribute to the program. The payments are transferred to the state, and federal Medicaid matching dollars are obtained. Then those hospitals in the state serving a disproportionate share of uncompensated care patients receive money from the new program. It is anticipated that statewide about 80 hospitals in the state will be eligible for disproportionate share payments through the program. The amount that a hospital contributes is based on its historic provision of MediCal and uncompensated care. The state expects to collect about $900 million this year and to return about $1.7 billion to the hospitals. For any particular hospital, the program will cover up to 80 percent of its annual uncompensated days.

New York has maintained a Bad Debt and Charity pool, which was established in 1983 to pay for uncompensated care. Under this arrangement, all hospital payers, except Medicare, contributed to the Pool. Disproportionate share payments were then made to hospitals from the pool on the basis of need. Until 1991, federal matching dollars were obtained only for those dollars Medicaid contributed to the pool. Then in 1991, New York "redefined" its disproportionate share program. In sum, the state shifted the entire Bad Debt and Charity Pool fund into Medicaid and began seeking federal matching dollars for all disproportionate share payments made in the state.

A large amount of money is involved in these programs. The Congressional Research Service estimates that in 1992, payments to providers related to provider tax and donation arrangements will amount to $11.4 billion, of which $6.9 billion are new federal funds. Disproportionate share payments, much of which are generated by provider taxes and donations, amounted to $16–18 billion in 1992. It should be noted that these mechanisms are more attractive the higher the federal matching rate. Since federal matching contributions are higher as a share of spending in poorer states, it is not surprising that provider tax and donation schemes have been more heavily used by low-income states. Since the low-income states were often the same states that were most affected by the pregnant women and children mandates, it seems that the mandates may have been financed much more with federal dollars than may be commonly realized.

This approach to creative financing is being limited. On December 12, 1991, the president signed into law the Medicaid Voluntary Contribution and Provider-Specific Tax Amendments of 1991. These amendments basically ban the use of donated funds as state matching funds and limit the use of provider-specific tax revenues to 25 percent of a state's total required match as long as the tax is applied on a broad basis. That is, the taxes must be uniformly imposed on all providers in a specific class. If a state, for example, continues to have a hospital tax, it must apply to all hospitals. In addition, the states are limited in the amount of Medicaid matching funds that will be available to pay disproportionate-share hospitals. Beginning in October 1992, a national and state limit on disproportionate share payments will be established. The national limit is set at 12 percent of total Medicaid expenditures. States that are currently above the limit must freeze it there, whereas those states not at the limit will be allowed to raise their disproportionate payment.

How states will be affected by these limitations is not known. If the states are able to broadly tax hospitals and nursing homes, they may continue to use this mechanism. In fact, in some states, the use of this approach could be expanded. For example, as of September 1991, only five states had exceeded the 25 percent cap (Alabama, Illinois, Kentucky, Maine, and Tennessee). Thirty states have not used provider taxes to obtain matching funds, so the new law still gives them the potential to increase their use of these mechanisms. The remaining states also have the potential to increase their matching funds under the new law. The constraint, however, is that taxes must be applied to all hospitals, not simply those serving Medicaid patients. There may be more potential to use provider taxes in nursing homes since Medicaid is the dominant payer in this market. The factor that may be more constraining to states is the 12 percent limit on disproportionate share programs since the national level already exceeds this level.

The use of provider donation and tax and disproportionate share arrangements has another implication. First, data on the level and rate of growth in Medicaid spending, both in total and at the state level, are overstated because of these transfers; only data on the increase in federal Medicaid spending are actually correct. One needs to subtract the contributions/taxes paid by hospitals and other providers that are in reality returned to them along with federal matching payments. Only the net spending actually reflects expenditures on Medicaid beneficiaries. Thus, data on Medicaid spending per enrollee are also inaccurate because some Medicaid dollars are also being used to finance some of the care provided to the medically indigent. Correspondingly, the number of people served by the Medicaid program is most likely understated since medically indigent persons are not typically counted as being Medicaid beneficiaries.

CONCLUSION

Medicaid spending has grown at extraordinary rates in recent years. This review of the data on the growth of spending shows that, unlike in prior years, Medicaid spending has grown faster than national healthcare spending on average, growing faster for adults and children than for the disabled and aged. The data support the argument that the large number of federal mandates has played an important role in explaining this growth. Mandates have been particularly important in the southern states, which have not been historically generous in covering their low-income populations. The increased coverage of these populations is likely to yield important benefits. To the extent that it results in a healthier low-income population, the benefits to society that will accrue at a later time will likely offset the costs.

But the mandates are only part of the story. There are a number of other reasons beyond the mandates for recent increases in Medicaid spending. First, the recession has increased Medicaid enrollment, particularly in the northeast but also in many other states. Second, inflation in health care costs has also been a major factor. Health care costs have increased for all payers, private and public. Medicaid programs are increasingly restrained by court decisions in keeping the rates of growth in spending below the growth rates of the market in general. Third, states have great difficulty in controlling spending on prescription drugs, a service that is increasingly costly to both public and private payers. Fourth, there has been an increase in demand for long-term care services. States have been successful in controlling nursing home spending, but have experienced a rapid growth in home health care.

Finally, the role of provider taxes and donations and disproportionate share programs has also contributed to the increases. Most of the states visited for this study have used provider tax and donation or disproportionate share arrangements to increase the level of federal financial participation in their programs. So, while mandates and other factors have had serious fiscal impacts on the states, they have not been as severe as they would have been if the states had not been creative in developing new financing mechanisms. The states would have had to have made highly unpopular cuts in their programs or would have had to more substantially restrict spending on other services if these mechanisms had not been employed. The use of provider tax and disproportionate share schemes, however, is playing a role beyond that of simply financing current benefits and reducing state outlays: It has permitted the states to use Medicaid to finance hospital uncompensated care. The beneficiaries of these new financing schemes include both hospitals and the medically indigent.

The Medicaid story of the past few years is one in which the states have come to clearly recognize the benefits of federal matching contributions. They have aggressively shifted a large number of the health and social services that they have provided to their populations into Medicaid. Thus, Medicaid has become a program to pay for health services for many of the uninsured, not simply those who are deemed categorically eligible for the program. This broadening of the Medicaid program is fundamental and has many implications, perhaps the most important being that the net additional cost to the federal government of a more rational approach to expanding care to the uninsured may be much less than has been previously realized.

REFERENCES AND NOTES

1. Reilly, T.W., Clauser, S.B., Baugh, D.K., "Trends in Medicaid Payments and Utilization, 1975–1989," *Health Care Financing Review, 1990 Annual Supplement.*

2. Department of Health and Human Services, Office of Management and Budget, *Better Management for Better Medicaid Estimates* (Washington, D.C., July 10, 1991).

3. These data are based on edited Health Care Financing Administration (HCFA) Form 2082 and Form 64 data for the fiscal years reported. These are reports filed by state Medicaid programs to describe program enrollees and services and to request federal matching dollars. The editing primarily consisted of adjusting expenditure data in Form 2082s to be consistent with the more accurate, but less disaggregated, expenditure data in the Form 64s.

4. Lazenby, H.C., and Letsch, S.W., "National Health Expenditures, 1989," *Health Care Financing Review* 12, no. 2 (Winter 1990).

5. Merlis, M., *Medicaid: Providing Donations and Provider-Specific Taxes* (Washington, D.C.: Congressional Research Service, October 2, 1991).

PART 2

.
.
.

Expanding Access and
Paying Providers

•

3

Medicaid Expansions and Access to Health Care

SARA ROSENBAUM

INTRODUCTION

This chapter reviews several of the most important federal Medicaid expansions enacted between 1984 and 1990. These expansions represent only a fraction of the scores of amendments adopted over the past decade but are representative of evolving Medicaid policy in the areas of primary, preventive, and acute (i.e., non-long-term care) services. A set of tables that sets forth the principal post-1980 Medicaid amendments appears in Appendix A of this volume.

Transforming a statutory behemoth like the Medicaid program takes far more than changing the law. Revisions to a statute the size and scope of Medicaid can take years to trickle down to the community level, where the impact of broad health policy reforms is ultimately measured. Only at this point can the true costs and benefits of reform be accurately measured.

It is important to remember that no statutory revision ever occurs in a vacuum. The Medicaid changes took place in the midst of a swirl of demographic, economic, and health care trends. These trends will influence their size, cost, and success. No matter how clearly a statutory goal has been articulated or how well the legislation has been drafted, in actual experience a program reform may work in ways that are completely different from what was anticipated. And the confounding events surrounding program implementation may make definitive cost estimation nearly impossible.

Nothing in Medicaid is ever simple. A seemingly straightforward statutory revision can (and has been) be interpreted in numerous ways by implementing federal agencies, states, and affected provider and beneficiary groups. Even simple changes can require extensive revision in federal and state policy and program operation equipment and materials, and the retraining of thousands of eligibility or claims payment staff at the state and local level.

Implementation has been further completed by the drawn-out process of enactment. Many of the reforms presented here as a single item were actually adopted through a lengthy series of legislative increments grafted onto annual budget-related bills. This piecemeal approach added to the confusion and difficulties faced in their implementation. In many cases, comprehensive legislation enacted all at once might have made the Medicaid reforms less costly to implement and more administratively humane. This did not happen, however, because of either actual or perceived political, ideological, or economic constraints. Ironically, many of these constraints ultimately may further increase costs by heightening inefficiencies and error rates.

Beyond the dilemma of determining the cost of reform is the challenge of deciding if *Medicaid* (as opposed to another type of programmatic) reform was the right route to follow in addressing a particular problem. For several reasons, during the 1980s, Medicaid became the legislative vehicle of choice. Some of the Medicaid initiatives, such as the federally qualified health center (FQHC) program, were ones that could not be developed through discretionary spending legislation because of the frequently severe spending constraints imposed on discretionary programs. Other reforms, such as the qualified Medicare beneficiary (QMB) program, were fashioned as Medicaid, rather than Medicare, expansions because of resistance to means rated premium assistance for Medicare beneficiaries.

To the extent that constrained discretionary health spending policies continue and fundamental alterations in public and private health insurance are not made, Medicaid probably will continue to play this "catch all" role—a role it has assumed for more than a quarter century. The program's relative structural elasticity and its multiple missions have made it a reasonably logical vehicle for reform. It remains to be seen whether the economy-tied constraints on state budgets and the new limitations on state options for financing their Medicaid programs (1) alter Medicaid's historic ability to "fill in the gaps."

This chapter examines six of the most important Medicaid expansions enacted since 1984, identifies the principal factors and intent underlying the expansions, and offers a preliminary assessment of the reforms' impact on both beneficiaries and the states. These six reforms, which include eligibility-related changes, benefit-related changes, and provider-related changes, are as follows:

Eligibility-related changes

1. Optional and mandatory coverage of poverty-level pregnant women and children;

2. Out-stationed enrollment for pregnant women, children, presumptive eligibility for pregnant women, and automatic coverage of newborns; and

3. The Qualified Medicare Beneficiary (QMB) program;

Benefit-related changes

4. The Early and Periodic Screening Diagnosis and Treatment (EPSDT) amendments;

Provider-related changes

5. Federally qualified health center services (including cost-based reimbursement for FQHCs); and

6. General obstetrical and pediatric provider payment reforms.

Their principal purposes were to expand eligibility, improve and ease the enrollment process, increase the scope and depth of covered benefits, increase provider reimbursement, and promote greater access to health services in areas designated as medically underserved by the United States Public Health Service.

Years later, it is still striking to consider how a decade that began with the election of a president who believed in reduced direct federal spending (and diminished mandated spending programs for the poor, in particular) could have concluded with unprecedented expansions in the most expensive of all poor people's entitlement programs. Over a six-year period, beginning in 1984, more than a half million pregnant women, between four and five million children, and millions of low income elderly and disabled Medicare beneficiaries were made eligible for Medicaid. Maternity and pediatric benefits were expanded, particularly in the case of children under age 21. The Medicaid enrollment process was fundamentally restructured in order to make access to coverage easier. The statute's provider reimbursement provisions were strengthened. In short, federal lawmakers altered virtually every feature that helps determine Medicaid's size and scope.

What makes these expansions even more notable is that the 1980s began with sweeping reductions in Medicaid (2). Benefits were effectively terminated for working poor women and children, and coverage requirements for other categories of children were curtailed. Legal requirements for coverage of medically indigent persons not eligible for cash assistance were down-scaled.

The Medicaid reforms that occurred during the latter part of the 1980s were striking because of the considerable political consensus on which so many were built. Between 1977 and 1980, a Democratic President and a Democratic Congress twice tried, and twice failed, to enact legislation covering only a portion of the pregnant women and children aided during the 1980s (3). Yet many of the most important program expansions for women and children were sought by federal lawmakers and governors of both parties, many of whom are better known for their cautious approach to expansion of federal direct spending generally and to entitlement growth

47

in particular. Indeed, the Medicaid expansions occurred even as real spending levels for other equally essential discretionary health and human service programs for the poor were allowed to erode significantly—a phenomenon that ironically directly helped justify several of the Medicaid expansions. By 1988, a Republican presidential candidate was campaigning on a health platform that included broad Medicaid expansions—a reflection of the political turnaround regarding Medicaid that had occurred in only seven years.

The Medicaid reforms also may have helped build a broader political and policy "tolerance level" for an expanded public third party financing program for the uninsured. Indeed, many of the financial, categorical, age-related, and other eligibility "cliffs" created by the recent reforms are perceived as unjust today, just as the lower cutoff points were judged a decade ago. As a result, a new generation of Medicaid proposals has been sponsored by Republicans and Democrats alike, who seek to improve Medicaid coverage for many of the persons left out in the first wave of reforms.

It may be impossible to accurately gauge the success or failure of reforms as complex as the six reviewed in this chapter. Most will take years to be fully implemented in terms of both cost and their impact on the health system for the poor. Furthermore, the world in which they are evolving is not static. Health insurance continues to erode. Poverty rates remain high. Health status measures remain depressed for significant segments of the American population. The cost of medical care continues to be uncontrolled. All of these factors will affect the ultimate size and scope of these changes.

Despite the measurable and non-measurable costs and burdens that many of the changes have imposed, it is fair to say that each reform reviewed here was enacted for a compelling reason. Many were widely supported by federal and state officials, as well as by beneficiary organizations. Some were adopted and implemented by states with historic speed. And virtually all, when fully implemented, will likely assist millions of the nation's poorest citizens. If the potential to help the poor is the best program measure available to policy makers for years to come, then the Medicaid reforms reviewed here should be considered a success.

ELIGIBILITY-RELATED REFORMS

Eligibility for pregnant women and children

Reform description

No fewer than seven times between 1984 and 1990 Medicaid was expanded to increase both optional and mandated coverage of low-income pregnant women and children ineligible for cash assistance benefits (4). The reforms, which are set forth in Table 1:

- require coverage of all pregnant women, infants, and children under age 6 with net family incomes not exceeding 133 percent of the federal poverty level and with resources not exceeding state-set standards (including the option to eliminate use of an asset test entirely) (5);

■ require coverage of all children born after September 30, 1983, who have attained age 6, who have not yet attained age 19, whose net family incomes do not exceed 100 percent of the federal poverty level and whose family assets do not exceed state set standards (including elimination of the asset test entirely) (5);

■ permit coverage, without use of an asset test, of pregnant women and infants under age 1 whose net family incomes do not exceed 185 percent of the federal poverty level; and

■ permit states to adopt more liberal standards and methodologies in determining net family income or resources for "poverty level" pregnant women and children (6) than those used under the cash assistance programs (7).

Table 1.

Medicaid Reform	Year of Enactment
Mandated coverage of single pregnant women, pregnant women in two-parent unemployed families, and all children born after 9/30/83 with AFDC-level income.	Deficit Reduction Act of 1984, P.L. 98-369
Mandated coverage of all remaining pregnant women with family income below AFDC eligibility levels and immediate coverage of all children under 5 with AFDC-level income.	Consolidated Omnibus Budget Reconciliation Act of 1985 P.L. 99-272
Optional coverage of all pregnant women and children born after 9/30/83 with family incomes not exceeding 100% of poverty and with family assets below state-set levels.	Omnibus Budget Reconciliation Act of 1986, P.L. 99-509
Optional coverage of pregnant women and infants with family incomes not exceeding 185% of poverty and family assets not exceeding state-set levels.	Omnibus Budget Reconciliation Act of 1987, P.L. 100-203
Mandated coverage of all pregnant women and infants with family incomes below 100 percent of poverty; option to use more liberal standards and methodologies.	Medicare Catastrophic Coverage Act of 1988, P.L. 100-360.

Table 1. (continued)

Mandated coverage of all pregnant women and children under age 6 with family incomes below 133% of poverty.	Omnibus Budget Reconciliation Act of 1989, P.L. 100-239.
Mandated coverage of all poverty level children under age 19 born after 9/30/1983 who have attained age 6 and with incomes up to 100% of poverty.	Omnibus Budget Reconciliation Act of 1990, P.L. 100-508.

Reform goals

The Medicaid maternal and child health reforms were enacted to improve poor women's and children's access to health services believed to enhance health outcome and have both short- and long-term cost effectiveness. They were enacted in the face of mounting evidence of rising childhood poverty and the loss of health insurance (8), as well as data from both official and non-governmental studies showing stagnation or erosion in such basic maternal and infant health indicators as prenatal care, low birthweight, infant mortality, and childhood immunization status (9).

Those reforms were sponsored by liberal and conservative lawmakers alike (10), and, when first enacted in optional form (in the case of coverage of poor pregnant women and children under age 5), received strong support from the nation's governors (11). The mandatory reforms ultimately enacted in 1989 and 1990 were essentially outlined by President Bush during his 1988 campaign (12).

Strong support came also from lawmakers opposed to abortion. During the 1970s many of these lawmakers had effectively blocked efforts to expand coverage for pregnant women and children by adding abortion restrictions to the Medicaid amendments when they were considered on the House floor. In the 1980s, however, with clear evidence of need and strong support from organizations known for their concern over both the well being of children and their opposition to abortion, many of these same lawmakers not only did not oppose the legislation but were actively involved in its passage (13). Passage was further aided by the fact that, with the exception of the mandates adopted in the Medicare Catastrophic Coverage Act (which provided its own shield), the maternal and child health reforms were insulated from political opposition by the larger budget reconciliation measures of which they were a part (14).

The cost of the legislation was probably underestimated, if only because it was unclear to most policy makers at the time of enactment how widespread child poverty had (and would continue to) become and how significant was the erosion of private insurance coverage. Moreover, probably only a handful of lawmakers anticipated the recession of the late 1980s, which swelled the numbers of women and children qualifying for Medicaid even under previous, more restrictive, coverage standards.

Impact on beneficiaries

The unforeseen costs growing out of the larger-than-expected numbers of women and children covered by an expanded Medicaid program are of course one measure of the expansion's success. Indeed, childhood poverty is now so high that if all states were to elect to cover all pregnant women and infants with family incomes below 185 percent of poverty, between 40 and 45 percent of all births in the United States potentially could be financed in whole or in part through Medicaid (15). As Table 2 shows, by 1992 more than half of all states had gone beyond the statutory minimum in coverage of pregnant women and infants. Seventeen states and the District of Columbia maintained income coverage rules for pregnant women and infants at the optional statutory level of 185 percent of poverty. Forty-seven states and the District of Columbia eliminated use of an asset test for poverty level pregnant women and children (16).

A 1991 telephone survey conducted by the Children's Defense Fund (CDF) to gauge the impact of the expansions offers further confirmation of their impact. In states in which Medicaid claims data could be matched against birth records, the CDF found that as many as 45 percent of all births were Medicaid financed. This represents a major increase over earlier estimates of the extent to which Medicaid finances births in the United States (17). The director of the Georgia Medicaid agency reported that in 1991 his program paid for nearly 60 percent of that state's births (18).

Not only are the absolute numbers of pregnant women receiving assistance through Medicaid high, but in numerous states, enrollment appears to closely approximate the pool of potentially eligible women—a degree of penetration that is virtually unprecedented. A 1991 Government Accounting Office (GAO) study found that within two years following the effective date of the 1986 maternity expansions for poor women, between two-thirds and three quarters of all estimated eligible pregnant women were enrolled. GOA officials also reported that, in several states, enrollment exceeded estimates (19).

From a beneficiary point of view, perhaps the most basic measure of success is that a "paper" benefit is in fact accessible. From this standpoint, the Medicaid reforms were highly successful; in fact, states responded so quickly to the 1986 coverage options that when coverage of poor women and children under age 6 was mandated in 1989, only seven states had not yet added coverage of poor pregnant women and infants, and only about half had not yet added coverage for at least some poor young children (20).

However strong the implementation of expanded maternity and infant coverage has been, there have been limits to the expansions' success that affect beneficiaries. First, unless a woman can qualify for Medicaid on some other basis (such as eligibility for AFDC), coverage is unavailable until her pregnancy is confirmed. This means that many women may go

Table 2. Medicaid coverage options for pregnant women and infants—July, 1992.

	PERCENTAGE OF POVERTY	EFFECTIVE DATE OF ORIGINAL EXPANSION
Alabama		Jul–88
Alaska		Jan–89
Arizona	140%	Jan–88
Arkansas		Apr–87
California	185%	Jul–89
Colorado		Jul–89
Connecticut	185%	Apr–88
Delaware	185%	Jan–88
DC	185%	Apr–87
Florida	185%	Oct–87
Georgia		Jan–89
Hawaii	185%	Jan–89
Idaho		Jan–89
Illinois	150%	Jul–88
Indiana		Jul–88
Iowa	185%	Jan–89
Kansas	150%	Jul–88
Kentucky	185%	Oct–87
Louisiana		Jan–89
Maine	185%	Oct–88
Maryland	185%	Jul–87
Massachusetts	185%	Jul–87
Michigan	185%	Jan–88
Minnesota	185%	Jul–88
Mississippi	185%	Oct–87
Missouri		Jan–88
Montana		Jul–89
Nebraska		Jul–88
Nevada		Jul–89
New Hampshire	150%	Jul–89
New Jersey	185%	Jul–87
New Mexico	185%	Jan–88
New York	185%	Jan–90
North Carolina	185%	Oct–87
North Dakota		Jul–89
Ohio		Jan–89
Oklahoma	150%	Jan–88
Oregon		Nov–87
Pennsylvania		Apr–88
Rhode Island	185%	Apr–87
South Carolina	185%	Oct–87
South Dakota		Jul–88
Tennessee	185%	Jul–87
Texas	185%·	Sep–88
Utah		Jan–89
Vermont	185%	Oct–87
Virginia		Jul–88
Washington	185%	Jul–87
West Virginia	150%	Jul–87
Wisconsin	155%	Apr–88
Wyoming		Oct–88
TOTAL	31	

Source: National Governors' Association, 1992.

through the crucial pre-pregnancy period in relatively poor health. Problems affecting their own health and that of their children go uncorrected and cannot be treated until well into pregnancy because of poverty and lack of health insurance (21).

A second limitation of the maternal and child health reforms is that many beneficiaries encounter major difficulties in locating sources of prenatal care unless they have access to a source of community health services for indigent persons such as those offered by local health departments or community health centers. Many of these programs have long waiting lists. Moreover, only a fraction of all communities in need of such programs have them at all (22).

The difficulties pregnant beneficiaries encounter in locating participating physicians have been captured in numerous studies of provider participation in Medicaid (23). The body of evidence on provider participation in Medicaid suggests that, once insured, many Medicaid-enrolled women continue to face major barriers to both primary and specialized care. These barriers appear to be significantly ameliorated only when Medicaid expansion strategies are combined with initiatives to increase the supply of services in medically underserved communities (24). Where this combined strategy has occurred, results have been significantly better than when Medicaid expansions alone are implemented (25).

A third problem is that as impressive as the rapid enrollment of pregnant women has been, there is some evidence that enrollment of eligible children has proceeded much more slowly. A far smaller proportion of eligible children appear to be enrolling in the program. This is true despite the fact that pregnancy and pediatric benefits were enacted in unison and despite widespread support for the pediatric eligibility expansions.

The number of children enrolled since enactment of the poverty expansions has been estimated at around 800,000 to 900,000 (26). It is unclear how many of these children are qualifying under the new standards or under the older, more restrictive standards. Anecdotal reports indicate some confusion around children's eligibility. For example, a survey of out-stationed enrollment programs at community health centers conducted by the CDF in late 1991 found that although the out-stationed Medicaid enrollment program (discussed later in this chapter) is required for both pregnant women and children, a number of centers reported no out-stationed services for children.

The newly eligible children, like their mothers, are most likely to be enrolled in Medicaid as a result of contact with the health care system. Unlike pregnant women, however, children (particularly poor and uninsured children and those beyond infancy) have fewer and more episodic health care contacts than pregnant women. They also have lower overall medical costs that may tend to diminish a family's sense of urgency in seeking help with medical bills, particularly if the family has a source of affordable care (such as a children's or public hospital outpatient clinic or a health center). Thus, there may be less likelihood that "older" children (i.e., those not identified through their mothers' receipt of prenatal care) will be identified in the absence of an aggressive outreach campaign aimed at locations other than health care clinics where poor children can be found. These locations are child care and Head Start programs, family service centers, and Food Stamp offices.

The lack of more rapid enrollment of eligible children is important because of the link between Medicaid coverage of poor children and their access to health care. Low-income children with Medicaid are significantly more likely than non-poor children to have a routine source of health care and are as likely as non-poor children to receive timely preventive health care, as shown in Tables 3 and 4. Indeed, the evidence on health care utilization among uninsured low-income children underscores Medicaid's impact on their access to health care.

Finally, the reforms appear to be having only marginal impact on particularly hard to reach children, such as those who live in migrant farmworker families. Anecdotal reports from some migrant health center directors suggest that when instituted, on-site enrollment programs work well in identifying Medicaid-eligible children. However, other center directors report that state failure to follow the special residency rules that pertain to migrant families and children (27), along with delays in the eligibility determination process and difficulties in documenting that eligibility criteria have been met, mean that very few eligible women and children are enrolled (28).

Impact on states

The maternal and child health eligibility reforms can be considered highly successful from a state implementation point of view. States adopted the optional reforms more swiftly than any other Medicaid option in the program's

Table 3. Percentages of children with usual source of care, under 18 years of age, in the United States, 1988.*

	Percentages of Children With Usual Source of Care by Type			
	Routine	Sick	Both Routine and Sick	Neither Routine nor Sick
All children†	90.5	93.3	87.8	4.6
Poor children‡	85.3	88.2	80.0	7.6
Without Medicaid	78.2	82.6	72.7	12.2
With Medicaid	90.9	92.7	85.8	4.0
Nonpoor children	92.1	94.9	90.0	3.5

*From microdata tapes from the 1988 National Health Interview Survey on Child Health.
†Includes data on children with unknown income or insurance status.
‡Includes data on children with unknown Medicaid status.
Source: St. Peter, R. F., Newacheck, P. W., and Halfon, N., "Access to care for poor children: Separate and unequal?" JAMA 267:20 (May 27, 1992).

Table 4. Percentages of children receiving routine care within recommended time interval, under 18 years of age, in the United States, 1988.*

| | Total Population | Usual Source of Routine Care | | | | |
		Physician's Office	Community Clinic	Hospital Clinic	Other	None
All children†	79.8	83.1	83.8	84.5	81.3	47.6
Poor children‡	77.5	81.4	84.8	84.0	78.2	50.5
Without Medicaid	69.2	75.4	75.9	71.7	79.2	45.5
With Medicaid	83.5	85.2	91.4	90.1	77.1	58.4
Nonpoor children	80.4	83.3	82.0	84.8	82.8	45.7

*From microdata tapes from the 1988 National Health Interview Survey on Child Health.
†Includes data on children with unknown income or insurance status.
‡Includes data on children with unknown Medicaid status.

Source: St. Peter, R. F., Newacheck, P. W., and Halfon, N., "Access to care for poor children: Separate and unequal?" *JAMA* 267:20 (May 27, 1992).

optional reforms more swiftly than any other Medicaid option in the program's history. There is simply no comparison between the state response to the options enacted during the mid-1980s and their response to earlier, more limited Medicaid coverage options for pregnant women and children.

For example, since 1965 states have had the option to cover all "financially needy" children under age 21 in families with AFDC-level income and resources (29). Beginning in 1967, states were given the option to cover all poor women with AFDC-level income (30). Less than a decade ago, when coverage for some of these children and pregnant women became mandatory, less than half of all states had in fact taken one or both options (31); even today, a minority of states cover all children under 21 in families with AFDC-level income.

The swiftness of the states' response is even more notable, given the fact that nearly six years after enactment of the first major optional reforms and two years after enactment of the last mandated reforms, there are still no current federal Medicaid eligibility regulations spelling out all statutory mandates and options with respect to coverage of children and pregnant women (or anyone else, for that matter). Unless one is intimately acquainted with the statute or is able to obtain and interpret the mass of federal Medicaid transmittals that periodically are sent to state Medicaid programs, there is no way to discern who must, and who may, be covered under Medicaid. While the statute is by and large self-enacting, its complexity is epic and the financial penalties for erroneous implementation are serious. There is no question that such quick state response to the eligibility options for pregnant women and infants is unique in Medicaid.

In sum, the potential impact of the reforms on pregnant women and children is great, given current high poverty levels and depressed access to private health insurance. The Medicaid expansions have extended eligibility for health insurance to hundreds of thousands of poor women and to millions of children who had virtually none. While enrollment rates for children remain a serious problem, in one sense expectations were unduly raised by the rapidity with which pregnant women were enrolled. Medicaid "take-up" rates for children—that is, the extent to which eligible children not receiving AFDC actually enroll in the program—traditionally has been estimated by the Congressional Budget Office (CBO) at approximately 50 percent. The CBO also commonly assumes at least five years before full program implementation levels are reached. But while it may be unrealistic to expect a more rapid enrollment rate, the need is very great and the cost of additional outreach is relatively modest.

From a state implementation perspective, the eligibility reforms were a success. The states responded to the reforms rapidly. Coverage of poor pregnant women and children, even on a mandated basis, is consistent with the Governors' recommendations over many years.

From a health outcomes perspective, it is too early to tell the degree of success achieved by the eligibility expansions. In the past, Medicaid expansions have been associated with infant mortality reductions and improvements in child health outcomes (32). Several recent studies also indicate that Medicaid eligibility reforms produce a measurable impact on infant mortality when implemented as part of an overall infant mortality reduction strategy that includes extensive outreach, expanded Medicaid eligibility, and greater Medicaid payment support for integrated health services programs operating in medically underserved communities (33).

These more recent studies suggest that Medicaid's importance in the area of maternal and child health may be dual in nature. It is both an individual entitlement that significantly improves access to primary and specialized outpatient and inpatient care as well as an important source of funding to support comprehensive health programs serving poor and uninsured patients. These programs' impact on child health has been documented. Medicaid coverage appears to have the most effect on child health outcome when service content and health care settings are carefully designed. Thus, it is important to future program reform efforts to continue to attend not only to basic coverage but also to benefit levels and program content and to the provider settings in which covered services are furnished.

This is a particularly appropriate time for research into the factors that make Medicaid an effective child health improvement tool. Medicaid agencies increasingly are becoming involved in the delivery of health services through the creation of managed care arrangements. If one of the central purposes of managed care is to assure access to effective health care, then further research into the attributes of a health care system that make the most difference to the health outcomes of very poor children is extremely timely.

Out-stationed enrollment, presumptive eligibility, and automatic newborn eligibility

Reform description

Out-stationed enrollment (OE), presumptive eligibility (PE), and automatic newborn coverage were added to the Medicaid statute in 1990, 1986, and 1984, respectively. Table 5 describes these reforms and their enactment. Both newborn coverage and PE have undergone further legislative revisions (once in the case of PE and twice in the case of newborn coverage) designed to improve their performance.

Automatic newborn coverage. The newborn coverage provision is a mandatory requirement that provides for automatic program enrollment of infants born to Medicaid-enrolled women. These infants are almost invariably eligible for coverage on their own, unless their family income pictures change dramatically. An analogy to the newborn coverage requirement is the automatic coverage rule for newborns without a waiting period, which virtually all states have adopted under their insurance laws.

Presumptive eligibility. Presumptive eligibility (PE), added to Medicaid in 1986, is an optional eligibility provision. It permits the states to extend temporary Medicaid coverage to pregnant women for ambulatory prenatal care while their applications are pending. The eligibility determination process can take months and cost valuable prenatal care time. Second, the PE program provides that PE application points be located at prenatal care sites where low-income women commonly receive services (e.g., WIC clinics, Title V–supported clinics, community and migrant health centers, and other state-financed prenatal care programs for low-income women). States have always had the option to out-station eligibility determination workers, but PE permits them to combine out-stationing with temporary coverage.

Third, PE allows the use of a very short application form and provides for on-site assistance to pregnant women applying for benefits. Fourth, PE assures temporary coverage, which lasts throughout the formal application period. It thus acts as an insurance "bridge," so that even if there are long application delays (a common occurrence in states with severe welfare agency staffing problems), pregnant women have a means to pay for prenatal care (34).

Out-stationed enrollment. The out-stationed enrollment (OE) program was enacted as a mandatory modification of the states' Medicaid application and eligibility determination procedures. Like PE, it provides for out-stationed enrollment at health clinics, but on a mandated basis. OE requires enrollment out-stationing for at least all poverty-level pregnant women and children applying for Medicaid. At a minimum, OE sites must be located at federally qualified health centers (FQHCs) and at disproportionate share hospitals. In order to cut down on length, states must use forms other than those used to enroll in the AFDC program. Finally, with the exception of the final eligibility determination itself (which under federal law can be performed only by a welfare agency employee) (35), the entire application process must occur at the OE site (36), thereby reducing travel time and beneficiary burdens.

Unlike PE, however, OE provides no temporary (i.e., "bridge") coverage during the application period. This means that unless states have elected to furnish PE coverage, pregnant women must wait until the application process has been completed before coverage begins. Moreover, even if PE is elected for pregnant women, children applying at OE sites can obtain no temporary coverage (although, as noted, infants do have automatic Medicaid coverage from birth).

Reform goals

The automatic, presumptive, and out-stationed reforms were designed to ease pregnant women's, infants' and children's enrollment into Medic-

Table 5. Automatic newborn coverage, presumptive eligibility, and outstationed eligibility.

Reform	Year of Enactment/Modification
Automatic newborn coverage: mandates automatic enrollment in Medicaid for one full year of infants born to women receiving Medicaid at the time of birth, so long as the infants remain with their mothers and so long as the mothers, if still pregnant, would remain eligible for Medicaid.	Deficit Reduction Act of 1984; amended in OBRA 1987 to require states to use mothers' Medicaid identifiers for infants pending issuance of separate identifier for infant. Amended again in OBRA 1990 to extend automatic newborn enrollment period from end of post-partum period (in the case of women losing Medicaid coverage after the post-partum period) to first full year of life.
Presumptive eligibility: optional state program that creates temporary eligibility for pregnant women pending formal eligibility determination process and out-stations the enrollment process at community prenatal care programs.	OBRA 1986; amended in Medicare Catastrophic Coverage Act of 1988 to add more classes of permissible PE providers; amended in OBRA 1990 to lengthen time periods for PE and for filing formal application for assistance.
Out-stationed enrollment: requires out-stationed enrollment for poverty-level pregnant women and children at FQHCs and DSH facilities, using simplified application forms.	OBRA 1990

aid and to avert delays in treatment. The mere fact of eligibility for Medicaid is not sufficient to assure that coverage actually reaches those who are entitled to it. Numerous studies have documented the barriers to Medicaid enrollment (37). These include long travel and waiting times, extensive application and eligibility verification requirements for both categorical and financial eligibility criteria (particularly verification of asset value) that impose burdens on both applicants and states (38), application forms that are in English only, and the general mismatch between entry points for health care for the poor and entry points for Medicaid.

Enrollment-related problems extend to eligibility redetermination as well. Many states redetermine eligibility in the case of Medicaid-only recipients on an annual basis (39). The redetermination process can impose the same burdens on beneficiaries, since the same level of paperwork is often required.

The barriers to Medicaid enrollment and retention have historically kept program participation rates well below estimated eligibility levels. Delays in application filing and processing also can contribute to the delayed onset of medical care. Even though providers serving persons determined eligible for coverage can be reimbursed retroactively for covered services rendered up to three months before the date of application, in fact many providers insist on evidence of valid and in-effect enrollment before rendering treatment.

While there is no quantitative evidence of the impact on provider access of not having evidence of actual Medicaid coverage in hand, an anecdote from the Mississippi Health Department illustrates the problem. Several years ago, health department officials reported the death of an infant in a small town. The baby's parents had applied for Medicaid for their child, but the child became ill while the family's application was still being processed. Although the family had a letter from the state agency indicating that the infant had been found eligible, no identification card had yet arrived. When the infant became extremely ill, the family sought care from numerous physicians, none of whom would see the baby without formal evidence of enrollment. The infant ultimately died before the card was ever issued.

Impact on beneficiaries

Anecdotal evidence from community health providers and state Medicaid agencies indicates that where it is in place, out-stationed enrollment through both OE and PE is enormously successful. Putting aside the confusion over OE assistance for children noted above, community health centers routinely report a near doubling of the proportion of potentially eligible persons actually enrolled in the program after out-stationing is instituted. Additionally, the Government Accounting Office (GAO) has concluded that out-stationing under the presumptive eligibility program was a key factor in the quick implementation of the pregnancy-related expansions (40). Out-stationing can assure application assistance to women and children and reduce enrollment barriers. It can also, when extended to include assistance during the redetermination process, limit the number of persons unnecessarily losing coverage (41).

Automatic newborn coverage should be of great value to beneficiaries as well, since it assures automatic coverage and bridges a critical period in a family's life. The program in effect helps assure health insurance coverage during the initial and confusing time period following an infant's birth.

Impact on states

By July 1991, 25 states and the District of Columbia were engaged in at least some out-stationing through adoption of the 1986 PE program. Thirty-one states had adopted a shortened Medicaid application, and 14 had expedited the application process for pregnant women (although many of these states did not have PE) (42).

In the case of OE, there have been both successes and confusion and resistance. At a 1992 meeting on OE sponsored by the National Governors Association, examples of strong state implementation efforts were highlighted. The program was credited with improving participation rates among pregnant women and children. However, a late Fall 1991 national survey of 300 federally qualified health centers conducted by the Children's Defense Fund found that only slightly more than 100 health centers had OE in place as described under the HCFA guidance and, moreover, that at some sites, OE assistance for children was not available (43). One of the major barriers to OE implementation appears to be confusion over whether states or health care providers are responsible for bearing the cost of the program. HCFA's written guidance (44) is ambiguous on this issue, although agency officials appear to take the position, at least orally, that OE is part of the Medicaid eligibility determination process itself and is therefore a state administration cost (45).

The automatic newborn program, while supported by many states, has had a long history of confusion. The 1984 amendments provided for automatic coverage of newborns but did not require states actually to provide newborns with Medicaid cards or other identifiers. An amendment was then added in 1987 to require states to permit providers to bill under the mother's identifier during the automatic coverage period. It was hoped that this would rectify the problem.

In 1990, however, when the automatic newborn program (which previously had been limited to the mother's period of Medicaid eligibility) was extended to a full year regardless of any change in the mother's coverage status, Congress again overlooked the identifier issue. Thus, it is now possible that many infants are "enrolled" in Medicaid but have no way to pay for care, because their mothers have lost their identifiers following the end of their 60-day post-partum coverage period.

There is no systematic information on how states are dealing with this problem. Anecdotal evidence indicates that at least some states appear to be making an effort to quickly issue cards for infants in order to reduce the time period during which they have no direct evidence of coverage. When asked, however, many health care providers are unaware that they can submit claims under mothers' identifiers in the case of infants under age one whose mothers are still enrolled in the program. In short, some eight years after initial enactment, there is apparently still widespread confusion around this important coverage issue for infants.

States appear to view the automatic newborn coverage provision as a positive measure. The 1990 newborn amendments to assure automatic enrollment for a full year regardless of the mother's eligibility status were sought by states themselves because of problems encountered in having infants "fall off" the program when their mothers' post-partum coverage period ended. However, the 1990 amendments did not succeed as envisioned. Their defeat represents a prime example of how a worthwhile and small (at least in the vast scheme of things) structural change to help beneficiaries can be defeated by very short-term budget concerns. As noted, the 1990 amendments were intended to guarantee uninterrupted enrollment for all babies born to Medicaid-enrolled women for 12 months. But the amendments were drafted ambiguously. The actual language of the statute provides for year-long automatic coverage for infants whose mothers, *if still pregnant, would qualify for coverage*. The plausible legal interpretation of this ambiguous language is that at the end of the mother's coverage period, her eligibility has to be redetermined, as if she were still pregnant. This redetermination provision obviously defeats the very purpose of the 12-month automatic enrollment amendment.

According to CBO and HCFA officials involved in the reforms, the amendments were apparently written ambiguously because of concerns over the potential added cost of clearly uninterrupted, year-long coverage for babies. In other words, budget estimators assumed that without aggressive enrollment procedures only a portion of eligible babies actually would receive coverage. Thus, changes to increase the number of babies actually enrolled and using services were treated as an additional program cost. Only those babies whose mothers could comply with a redetermination requirement— the very barrier Congress had sought to eliminate—were assumed as continuously enrolled for 12 months. Removing this redetermination barrier would mean that more babies would actually stay in the program beyond the post-partum period and use benefits. Thus, an amendment that the states themselves sought in order to improve program performance for infants was effectively stopped over a nearly insignificant amount of additional federal spending given the overall magnitude of the Medicaid program.

HCFA guidance implementing the 1990 amendments does give the states the option to waive the redetermination requirement for mothers. But at the time of the issuance, several state Medicaid officials indicated that they would have trouble convincing their budget offices to accept this option because the CBO's assumptions of potential cost and because they were required not to take any options that could increase program costs.

Qualified Medicare Beneficiaries

Reform description

The Qualified Medicare Beneficiary (QMB) program was mandated as part of the Medicare Catastrophic Coverage Act to assure that indigent Medicare beneficiaries would be shielded against higher premium costs. It was again expanded in the Omnibus Budget Reconciliation Act of 1990 to protect near-poor beneficiaries against rising Medicare Part B premium costs.

The QMB program requires state Medicaid programs to pay Medicare premiums, deductibles, and copayments for elderly and disabled Medicare beneficiaries with annual incomes up to 100 percent of the federal poverty level in 1992. By 1995 the QMB program is scheduled to cover all Medicare beneficiaries with incomes up to 120 percent of the federal poverty level. An asset limit of $4,000 for QMB individuals and $6,000 for QMB couples is also imposed.

The QMB amendments also require state Medicaid programs to pay the Medicare cost-sharing requirements for elderly and disabled Medicare beneficiaries poor enough to qualify for full Medicaid coverage. Prior to enactment of the QMB amendments, many states had paid Medicare cost-sharing for their "dual enrollees" (that is, Medicare beneficiaries also entitled to Medicaid) as a means of cost-savings. For benefits covered by both programs, Medicare is the primary payer.

Reform goals

The mandatory QMB reforms were enacted in order to shield low-income Medicare beneficiaries financially ineligible for Medicaid (46) from the heavy burden of out-of-pocket payments resulting from both the cost-sharing requirements under the Medicare program. These burdens exacerbate an already serious out-of-pocket burden on low-income Medicare beneficiaries arising from Medicare's coverage limitations (47). While states have had the option since 1986 to extend full Medicaid coverage (not simply Medicare cost-sharing protections) to poor elderly and disabled persons, only a tiny number have done so. The QMB protections assure that low-income, Medicaid-ineligible, elderly and disabled persons at least can conserve their limited disposable resources for medical care not covered by Medicare (such as prescribed drugs, dental care, eyeglasses, and so forth).

As significant as the out-of-pocket burden under Medicare has been historically, it became far more so with passage of the 1988 Medicare Catastrophic Coverage Act. The Act substantially expanded Medicare benefits but also increased cost-sharing requirements. Even after the Act was repealed, Medicare cost-sharing burdens remained high, particularly with the Medicare deductible increase, which was enacted as part of OBRA 1990 (48).

A study conducted by Families USA found that from 1980 to 1992, total

Medicare Part A and Part B deductible and premium costs rose by more than 230 percent (49). These uncovered costs alone amount to nearly 25 percent of a single, poor Medicare beneficiary's 1992 annual income. Moreover, these out-of-pocket costs do not include the cost of uncovered care or the cost of uncovered copayments or allowable balance billing by providers. Thus, low-income Medicare beneficiaries can remain uninsured against not only care and services not covered by Part B, but by Part B–covered services as well, for they cannot pay program premiums.

Impact on beneficiaries

The Families USA study found that the QMB program had enrolled only 47 percent (slightly more than 2 million persons) of the estimated 4.2 million non-institutionalized elderly Medicare beneficiaries meeting the QMB eligibility criteria (50). Moreover, the 2 million enrollment figure appears to include all elderly non-institutionalized Medicare buy-in recipients, including elderly persons eligible for the buy-in because they are eligible for full Medicaid coverage as well (51). Thus, the true penetration rate for the non-Medicaid eligible QMBs may be lower (52).

As noted above, a 50 percent enrollment rate is not necessarily unduly low for a Medicaid-only coverage program. In general (and with the important and apparent exception of pregnant women in many states), many persons eligible for Medicaid are missed. But the QMB enrollment arrangement poses particular difficulties for the elderly poor. QMB benefits directly compensate for Medicare's cost-sharing deficiencies and indirectly compensate its coverage limitations. But obtaining the benefits requires filing a separate Medicaid application at a local welfare office, not at the Social Security Administration where Medicare claims are handled. The additional travel and application time poses a major barrier to elderly enrollment. There is no mandated out-stationed enrollment program for QMBs at community health centers, physicians' offices, hospitals, or other sites where the poor elderly receive medical care, as is the case with pregnant women and children. Nor is there a presumptive eligibility program that permits cost-sharing assistance to begin as soon as a preliminary determination of QMB eligibility is made.

Given the relatively simple nature of the information needed to establish QMB eligibility, mail-in applications might also be possible. However, there do not appear to be mail-in QMB programs. As of March 1992, according to Families USA, HCFA had no routine system for mailing notices to Medicare beneficiaries about the availability of the QMB benefit or where and how to obtain benefits.

Impact on states

The governors have been extremely unhappy with the QMB program, although state agencies themselves have sought improvements in the structure and scope of the QMB program (53). In March 1991, the National Governors Association called for repeal of the QMB benefit. The governors have consistently taken the position that the financial medical burdens that fall on the elderly and disabled poor as a result of the shortcomings of Medicare are the responsibility of the federal government, although in other contexts they have supported Medicaid coverage of all poor persons, even those with some limited health insurance coverage through other sources (54).

Beyond general dissatisfaction with QMB, some states also have sought to limit their QMB exposure by limiting their coverage of Medicare copayments to only those Part B services for which Medicare payments do not meet or exceed the state's Medicaid fee. At least one state has been successfully sued over this "cross-over claims" issue, which can leave both poor Medicare beneficiaries and health care providers with substantial amounts of uncovered expenses. HCFA has taken the position that states need not pay the Part B copayment in these situations and has even indicated that no copayment might be needed in cases in which the state's Medicaid reimbursement level actually exceeds the amount which Medicare pays (55).

Ideally, given the barriers elderly and disabled Medicare beneficiaries confront in having to make separate applications for Medicaid in order to obtain Medicare cost-sharing assistance, the financial help embodied in the QMB program would come as an integral part of the Medicare program. Short of that, the QMB program might be better integrated with Medicare. A fully integrated Medicare/Medicaid QMB system might enroll elderly beneficiaries at Social Security offices or at out-stationed provider sites or by mail.

In the absence of this integration, and without clearly delineating the "new" QMBs from the Medicaid-enrolled QMBs, it is extremely difficult to say how financially burdensome the QMB legislation is. As noted above, for years most states have paid Medicare Part B premiums for their Medicare-eligible populations, precisely because it is cost effective to do so. The marginal cost of buying into Medicare for non-dually eligible Medicare beneficiaries might well be offset by their improved access to medical care and their reduced need for Medicaid to pay for high-cost illnesses.

BENEFIT-RELATED REFORMS

The Early and Periodic Screening Diagnosis and Treatment (EPSDT) Amendments of 1989

Reform description

In 1989 the EPSDT program—special medical assistance benefits for all Medicaid enrolled children under age 21—was substantially revised and expanded. The principal reforms required states to:

- adopt medically reasonable periodic well-child screening schedules that comport with accepted standards of medical and dental practice;

- provide children with "interperiodic" screens (e.g., examinations on an as-needed basis, even if in between regularly scheduled screens) whenever a problem is "suspected";

- pay for all medically necessary care falling within the federal definition of medical assistance (56) for children whose periodic or interperiodic screens reveal one or more problems, even if such services are not covered for persons over age 21 or are not provided in the same amount, duration and scope.

Reform goals

The 1989 EPSDT amendments represent a potentially significant expansion of the special pediatric benefit package to which all Medicaid beneficiaries under age 21 have been entitled since 1967. Depending on the extent of the states' coverage limitations in effect prior to 1989, the reforms add some, or many, services for children or broadly expand the amount, duration, and scope of services that are covered. Moreover, the reforms require that expanded services be covered *whenever* a need arises, not just at periodic intervals, as under prior law. Thus, in some states, the *frequency* of children's access to comprehensive coverage has been greatly enhanced.

The 1989 reforms represented an attempt to deal with EPSDT's longstanding incongruities and deficiencies. These shortcomings arise out of EPSDT's disconnected relationship to the basic pediatric Medicaid program. Historically, EPSDT screening and treatment benefits were available only at periodic "well-child" intervals. The interperiodic screening and treatment amendments essentially did away with EPSDT as simply a separate well-child program. Expanded EPSDT assessment and treatment benefits are now covered for children regardless of whether their health care encounter is for a regularly scheduled, routine check-up or a suspected medical problem or condition. Whether the amendments will achieve this deeper goal of integrating EPSDT into basic Medicaid policy for children will not be known for some time, however. States are still in the midst of revising their programs to meet the new requirements and HCFA has, as yet, issued no formal rules (57).

To understand the magnitude of, and the intent behind, the 1989 amendments, some program background is helpful. EPSDT was created in 1967 and had two missions. The first, embodied in the *Medicaid* EPSDT amendments, was to add coverage for preventive health care for children under 21, even if such services were not covered for adults. The second, embodied in a *separate set of* amendments to the Title V Maternal and Child Health Services program, was to assure that state maternal and child health agencies would actively seek out, screen, and treat poor children, including Medicaid-eligible children. Congress envisioned that state Medicaid agencies would pay for services furnished by Title V agencies (58).

From its inception, the Medicaid EPSDT amendments required the states to pay for periodic health exams (i.e., screens) to determine the existence of health problems. EPSDT rules promulgated in 1971 also required the states to pay for immunizations and vision, dental, and hearing services and any other medical care treatment needed to correct health problems disclosed during a periodic screen, so long as the treatment was otherwise covered under the state's Medicaid plan (59). The states could deny coverage for assessment and treatment services furnished "interperiodically" (that is, in between the regularly scheduled screening intervals) and could also deny coverage for needed care not otherwise included in their plans for adults.

Thus, despite the importance of the program in the areas of well-child exams, immunizations, and vision, dental, and hearing care, EPSDT's reach was limited. Children could not get care on an "as-needed" basis, and those with more costly and chronic medical conditions found that many types of care and services (such as mental health services) were uncovered.

From the beginning the EPSDT program, even in its more limited state, generated much controversy and numerous efforts designed to force states to provide children with more frequent—and more—EPSDT screens. After extensive federal and state implementation delays (60), Congress enacted legislation in 1972 penalizing the states for their failure to inform children of EPSDT and furnish timely services if requested (61). A financial penalty equal to a one-percent reduction in federal AFDC payments was to be imposed. *Low numbers of provider claims for EPSDT screening services in comparison to the number of children requesting EPSDT services were considered evidence of children's poor access to preventive health care generally.* The 1972 amendments in effect placed service provision responsibilities directly on state Medicaid agencies rather than on Title V programs and thus represented a major departure from Medicaid's role as a service payer rather than a service assurer. Suddenly, Medicaid agencies found themselves responsible for assuring that care was furnished, not simply paid for (62).

There were numerous lawsuits to enforce states' "AFDC penalty" outreach and screening obligations. An early case resulted in a sweeping victory that underscored the preventive nature of the program and required the state Medicaid agency to take aggressive steps to find and screen children (63). Others resulted in settlements in which states agreed to institute outreach programs. Still other cases failed because plaintiffs were unable to prove that children were in fact not obtaining preventive health exams (64) or that states' outreach efforts (most often written materials distributed at the time of welfare application) were insufficient.

In these cases there invariably was evidence that high numbers of families were in fact not requesting EPSDT services. Advocates attributed the failure to request services to poor informing. The states attributed these low numbers to the fact that parents already were receiving preventive health care for their children and therefore did not need EPSDT screens. However, other lawsuits brought during this time period successfully challenged states' failure to cover adequate levels of services (particularly dental coverage limitations) for children who did request EPSDT (65).

In 1981 the "penalty statute"was repealed (66). However, the program's informing and service requirements were codified directly into the "state plan" provisions of the Medicaid statute (67).

Thus, the focus of the program remained on measuring the scope and quality of the states' pediatric health care programs by counting the number of provider screening claims forms. States that did not use EPSDT-specific claims forms, and states that paid for preventive health care as both an EPSDT and a general Medicaid service, continued to protest this claims form measure as a highly inaccurate proxy of children's access to preventive health care.

The use of inaccurate performance measures continued to be the issue of the extent to which Medicaid children were already receiving preventive health care—and how much they received (68).

More recent research into utilization of health services by Medicaid children indicate that the states were right in pointing out the inaccuracy of the EPSDT claims form as a measure of access to preventive health services. Studies show that Medicaid-enrolled children, unlike uninsured children, do, in fact, receive preventive health services. Table 4 shows that more than 90 percent of all Medicaid-enrolled children have a regular source of health care and receive timely preventive health services (69). On the other hand, only about 25 percent of all Medicaid-enrolled children receive EPSDT screens. Clearly, therefore, EPSDT screening claims forms tell only a portion of the story when it comes to children's use of preventive health services.

But while the states were correct in pointing to the insufficiency of the EPSDT screening form as a measure of use of preventive health care, serious general problems remained. Many providers furnishing preventive health care to Medicaid children omit crucial elements of the EPSDT program, particularly developmental assessments, immunizations, and lead toxicity screens. Moreover, the structure of EPSDT meant that children could obtain EPSDT services only periodically and that many conditions potentially could go untreated for lack of coverage.

The 1989 EPSDT amendments were an attempt to assure Medicaid coverage for all necessary health care whenever it is needed. As a result, EPSDT is, in effect, no longer a separate program (although EPSDT informing still remains an obligation, and the statute now requires specific reporting on EPSDT screening rates). It is now a broad bundle of comprehensive benefits that are available whenever children need them. Given the "unbundling" of EPSDT, it thus makes more sense to test the effectiveness of the states' pediatric programs through more careful monitoring for the provision of *specific services* that pediatric providers commonly do furnish. For example, if lead screening is a service that physicians commonly will not perform, the states might be assessed for the alternative steps they have taken to work with other agencies to develop and pay for aggressive lead testing and treatment programs in high-risk communities. Similarly, if physicians resist immunizing children because of low payment rates and fears of malpractice (70), then HCFA should assess the alternative steps state agencies are taking to assure access to and payment for immunization services. In other words, since it is now understood that counting screens does not accurately depict a state's program, the choices are to either develop a more reliable reporting instrument or monitor for particularly common service omissions by providers.

Impact on beneficiaries

The 1989 amendments represent a major expansion of the program for children. Particularly lacking in many states has been coverage of services needed by children at risk for chronic mental health and developmental disabilities and delays (71). By requiring treatment as needed and coverage of all possible forms of permissible "medical assistance," the amendments open up new service possibilities, including broader coverage and additional service settings to the extent permitted under federal law.

Impact on states

The EPSDT amendments caused great concern on the states' part because of the potential magnitude of the new benefit requirements. Moreover, although the overall intent of the amendments was to expand benefits and reduce the reliance on periodic EPSDT screens alone as a measure of state program performance, the retention of an EPSDT screening target rate for the states undermined this move away from counting screens as a proxy for state performance. In 1991 the National Governors Association called for the repeal or modification of the EPSDT amendments.

It will take a long time, and carefully designed studies will be required, to determine the actual impact of the amendments. In states with relatively generous coverage levels, the benefit expansions will have only a very modest impact. In states with limited coverage, the amendments may have a greater impact on state *Medicaid* budgets. But offsets to other state health budgets for children (particularly savings to state special education programs, Title V programs for children with special health care needs, and developmental disability and mental health programs) must be taken into account in order to determine the amendments' additional actual cost.

Over 12 million children now are eligible for expanded Medicaid services. Compared to non-poor children, a disproportionate number will need specialized treatment (although the vast majority probably will never need many of the specialized services states were required to add). Certainly all states will experience at least some costs as they implement the reforms, and that total cost will probably be far higher than the amount estimated by CBO staff (who did not take into account the new inter-periodic program). But the true cost of the reforms will not be known for many years and probably can be discerned only through careful, cross-program study.

PROVIDER-RELATED REFORMS

The federally qualified health centers amendments and provider reimbursement reforms of general applicability

Reform description

In 1989 Congress added two important provider provisions to the statute. The first was incorporation into the statute of a long-standing federal regulation governing sufficiency of provider reimbursement. The second was the creation of the federally qualified health centers (FQHC) program, modeled after the long-standing Medicare federally funded health centers (FFHC) program and the 1977 Medicare/Medicaid rural health clinic services act (72).

The sufficiency of payment provision. The sufficiency of payment statute, like its regulatory predecessor, requires states to establish provider reimbursement levels sufficient to assure beneficiaries reasonable access to care (at least to the extent that such care is available to the general population of a given geographic area). In addition, the 1989 amendments established specific state plan requirements governing payment for obstetric and pediatric services. Under the amendment, obstetric services include services furnished by obstetricians and family practice physicians, as well as the services of mid-level practitioners such as nurse midwives and nurse practitioners. Pediatric services include the services of family practice physicians, pediatricians, and mid-level practitioners. Inpatient services and institutional services were not included in the special reporting requirements, although, like all Medicaid services, the care and services of institutional providers are covered by the general sufficiency of payment requirement.

States must furnish HCFA with specific information showing that their payments to these two classes of providers are sufficient. This may be shown, under HCFA guidance, by demonstrating either that rates are reasonable in relation to private charges or that there is a sufficient number of providers participating "fully" in Medicaid.

The FQHC amendments. The FQHC amendments did three things. First, they created a new class of Medicaid providers known as federally qualified health centers. As noted above, this provider class was modeled after the 25-year-old FFHC program. However, FQHCs include not only all federally funded community and migrant health centers (as was the case under the older FFHC program) but also health care programs for the homeless funded under the Stewart McKinney Homelessness Assistance Act, entities (known as "look-alikes") (73) that meet the funding requirements of the three programs, and outpatient health programs operated by Indian tribes or tribal organizations under the Indian Self-Determination Act. In addition, entities applying for FQHC "look-alike" status may receive waivers of certain federal FQHC certification requirements for up to two years (74).

Thus, the entities that qualify as FQHCs may go well beyond the approximately 600 federally funded health centers. The purpose of this new provider definition was to assure adequate payment to a wide variety of community-based public and private non-profit entities funded with grants and furnishing primary health care on an income-adjusted basis. Members of Congress (particularly those with large numbers of non-federally funded health centers in their states) (75) believed that entities that make primary health care available to the uninsured should be assured of Medicaid (and Medicare) payments that cover their reasonable costs. Congress desired to avoid cost-shifting onto grants because of what this meant for the provision of uncompensated care to low-income uninsured persons.

Second, the FQHC amendments require that the states pay for certain care and services FQHCs furnish, regardless of whether those services are paid for when furnished by other providers (76). This special mandated bundle of care and services is known as "FQHC services." For example, FQHC services include services of clinical psychologists and social workers, even if these practitioners' services are not covered when offered in other outpatient service settings.

Third, the amendments require that FQHCs be paid on a reasonable cost basis for the "FQHC" services they furnish, as well as for any other ambulatory service they furnish that is covered under the state Medicaid plan (77).

Reform goals

The payment sufficiency reforms were added to the statute in an effort to raise provider reimbursement rates generally. They were also designed to assure that the states took specific steps to more adequately compensate for pediatric and obstetrical services. They reflect an enormous body of information on the depressed level of Medicaid provider fees generally (78).

By requiring specific information on provider fee levels and participation in the case of obstetrics and pediatrics, Congress hoped that it would learn more about fees paid for pediatric and obstetrical care and lay the basis for further provider payment reform. While Members of Congress also hoped that higher fees would encourage greater participation, it was generally assumed that even with substantial participation increases, provider access problems would remain. However, Congress believed that without clear statutory sufficiency of payment requirements and ongoing data collection, further improvements would be difficult.

The FQHC amendments were enacted for several reasons. First, there was widespread congressional concern that health centers and other similar programs were being forced to use declining federal, state, local, and private grants meant for the care of the uninsured to offset Medicaid reimbursement rates that covered less than their reasonable cost of operation. Second was congressional recognition of the importance of Medicaid revenues to health center support. When the health centers program was first created in 1965, HEW officials anticipated that 80 percent of their operating revenues would come from Medicare and Medicaid, with grants used to support only remaining uncovered costs and as working capital to expand or create programs. The 1989 amendments represented further steps to assure adequate third-party payment support for health centers and similar programs.

Third, the FQHC amendments reflect congressional recognition of the importance of health centers to the communities they serve. By law, centers are located in only the most severely medically underserved inner-city and rural communities. Even if Medicaid fees were increased, many, if not most, of these communities would continue to have trouble attracting sufficient physicians. Moreover, studies suggest that even sizable fee increases, while associated with an increase in Medicaid participation rates, do not assure sufficient participation by community physicians to obviate the need for additional efforts to create a better supply of providers (79). Congress viewed additional financial support for health centers as a means of helping them attract and retain medical and professional staff, upgrade services, establish new locations, and so forth.

Finally, the FQHC amendments were supported by numerous studies which, while older, show that health centers are effective in improving community health (80).

Impact on beneficiaries

Clearly one of the most troubling aspects of Medicaid for beneficiaries has been the lack of providers willing to participate in the program or available to treat patients. To the extent that provider fee increases improve Medicaid participation, the sufficiency reforms are extremely important. And to the extent that the FQHC reforms permit health centers and other entities serving the poor to see more patients, expand locations, or recruit or retain more providers with their increased revenues, patients are well served.

Impact on the states

As of 1992, approximately two thirds of all states had received plan approval for their pediatric and obstetric sufficiency plan amendments.

Approximately one third had state plan amendments disapproved for failure to show either that rates were adequate or, alternatively, that there were enough providers available in all geographic areas.

In the case of FQHCs, by the end of 1991 (more than a year after the amendments' effective date) only 24 of 32 surveyed states in one study had begun to pay centers on a reasonable cost basis and only 15 included payment for all ambulatory services in their reasonable cost rates (81). Moreover, only a small portion of states paying interim cost-based rates had begun the reconciliation process to assure that all reasonable costs were in fact reimbursed.

The states have expressed a great deal of unhappiness with the FQHC program, although the general sufficiency requirements appear to have caused little concern (perhaps because the statute simply codifies long-standing regulatory requirements). The states believe that the cost-based FQHC rate is a subsidy for the inadequate funding levels provided by the federal government under the federal health centers program. Many states also believe that the retrospective, cost-based FQHC payment methodology runs counter to preferred payment mechanisms, such as negotiated rates or capitated payments.

The states' concerns over payment of additional subsidies to health centers are much like their concerns over the Medicare QMB program—namely, that the program compensates for failures in the federal health policy arena.

Moreover, the states are extremely concerned over the FQHC "look-alike" program or, more specifically, the "waivered look-alike" program. As noted above (82), the "true" look-alikes (i.e., those entities that meet all federal health center funding requirements) represent only a fraction of the certified FQHCs to date. Far more numerous are entities that do not meet FQHC standards. The decision by HCFA and the Public Health Service to grant waivers for such items as 24-hour coverage, hospital linkages, and other absolutely essential features of the community health centers program calls into serious question whether the purpose of the FQHC statute—building comprehensive care in underserved areas—is being frustrated. Thus, while the size of the total look-alike program is small to date, waivered look-alikes dominate the landscape. The practice of granting waivers of essential health center characteristics such as 24-hour coverage and hospital admission arrangements should be considered quite serious.

Both the general provider sufficiency requirements and the FQHC provisions are far too new to reliably gauge their successes and costs. To the extent that provider reimbursement increases add physicians and obstetricians to the program in appreciable numbers, the added payments may well be considered worth their cost. And to the extent that enhanced FQHC revenues are used to increase the total number of patients served, add staff or services, increase the scope of operations and locations, or make other important patient care reforms, they will be successful. How the added FQHC funds are being invested and the amount of the funds actually attributable to the heightened reimbursement levels (as opposed to revenue increases arising from expanded eligibility) represent important items for further research.

CONCLUSION

Much research is needed over the coming years to evaluate the costs and effectiveness of the reforms described here. None of the reforms was adopted for less than compelling reasons. Many build on long-standing provisions of the statute and have deep roots in prior Medicaid policy. Whether the reforms succeed as planned will help determine the shape of future Medicaid reform and health care financing reforms generally. And for the millions of beneficiaries whose access to health care would be far more constrained without Medicaid, the expansions discussed in this chapter hold the promise of more affordable and better health care.

REFERENCES AND NOTES

1. The Medicaid Moratorium Amendments of 1991 place new limitations on states' historically broad discretion in generating their Medicaid program funding. The amendments restrict the use of certain types of dedicated taxes and place upper limits on the revenues that can be generated from even lawful forms of dedicated taxes. The amendments potentially force states to finance a greater share of their programs out of general revenues, which are already badly squeezed by competing state and community needs.

2. See Appendix A, which identifies the Medicaid-related reductions.

3. The Child Health Assurance Act passed by the House of Representatives in 1979 would have extended Medicaid to children under 18 with family incomes under 66 percent of the federal poverty level and to pregnant women with family incomes under 80 percent of the federal poverty level. Federal mandatory eligibility standards are now far higher.

4. Expansions were also enacted for women of childbearing age and children *no longer eligible for* aid for families with dependent children (AFDC) payments. Four months of extended benefits were enacted for women and children losing AFDC because of increased spousal and child support, and 12 months' additional coverage was provided for families losing AFDC because of increased earnings. 42 U.S.C. §1396r-6 and §1396t (1992).

5. 42 U.S.C. §1396a(a)(10)(A) and §1396a(l) (1992).

6. This is the name collectively given to pregnant women and children whose eligibility is based on financial need alone.

7. Eligibility for Medicaid depends on families' net, rather than gross, income. Under this option, states can adopt more generous deductions in determining net income for Medicaid eligibility purposes than would be used for determining AFDC eligibility. For example, the AFDC program limits child care deductions of approximately $200 per month. In determining Medicaid eligibility, however, states can take into account all necessary child care

expenses. This means that children in families with gross incomes well above 133 percent of poverty may nonetheless be entitled to Medicaid.

8. See, e.g., U.S. Bipartisan Commission on Health Care, *A Call for Action* (Washington, D.C., 1990); National Commission on Children, *Beyond Rhetoric* (Washington, D.C., 1990); Institute of Medicine, *Preventing Low Birthweight* (Washington, D.C.: National Academy Press, 1985); National Commission to Prevent Infant Mortality, *Death Before Life* (Washington, D.C., 1988); Children's Defense Fund, *The Health of America's Children* (Washington, D.C., 1986, 1987, 1988, 1989, 1990, 1991); White House Task Force on Infant Mortality, *Preliminary Report* [Unpublished] (Washington, D.C., 1989); Congressional Research Service, *Children in Poverty* (Washington, D.C., 1984); Children's Defense Fund, *American Children in Poverty* (Washington D.C., 1984).

9. See, e.g., Institute of Medicine, *Preventing Low Birthweight* (Washington, D.C.: National Academy Press, 1985); National Commission to Prevent Infant Mortality, *Death Before Life* (Washington, D.C., 1988); Alan Guttmacher Institute, *Blessed Events and the Bottom Line* (Washington, D.C., 1987); Food Research and Action Center, *The Widening Gap* (Washington, D.C., 1984); Children's Defense Fund, *The Health of America's Children* (Washington, D.C., 1985, 1986, 1987, 1988, 1989, 1990, 1991).

10. Legislation to expand Medicaid for children was co-sponsored by Republican and Democratic lawmakers in 1985, 1986, 1987, 1988, and 1989. For additional information, readers should consult the legislative histories to the various bills incorporated into the legislation that appears in Appendix A of this volume.

11. In 1984, the Southern Governors Association, led by then So. Carolina Governor Richard Riley, established a special infant mortality project, whose mission was to reform Medicaid to cover women and children more broadly as part of a comprehensive infant mortality reduction and child health strategy. The project issued several reports and was highly instrumental in convincing the Southern Governors Association and ultimately, the National Governors Association, to support passage in 1986 of Medicaid coverage options for all poor pregnant women and children under age 5.

12. See, Bush Election Campaign, *Invest in Our Children* (Washington, D.C., 1988).

13. The elimination of Medicaid funding for abortion as an issue in maternal and child health expansion legislation probably is the result of several factors. First, the budget reconciliation vehicles that came to house the child health expansions were vast, "must-do" pieces of legislation that were not considered appropriate legislative vehicles for non-budget-related, politically controversial social reforms. Second, the House Select Committee on Children, formed in 1982 and whose membership included several key members with strong anti-abortion positions, spent several years developing strong support from its members for the reforms. These Select Committee members in turn convinced other anti-abortion Representatives not to introduce limiting amendments. Third, the United States Catholic Conference provided strong support, a critical factor in convincing pro-life members to refrain from offering anti-abortion riders to the legislation.

14. The Budget Act Agreement of 1990 effectively did away with the budget reconciliation process during the five-year period in which the agreement is in effect. The Medicaid Moratorium Amendments of 1991 are evidence that

Medicaid reduction legislation will proceed without a reconciliation vehicle. Whether expansion measures can also proceed remains to be seen.

15. This estimate is based on an unpublished report by the White House Task Force on Infant Mortality which, in 1989, reported that 45 percent of all births in the United States are to women with family incomes below 200 percent of the federal poverty level. Since the 185 percent eligibility test for pregnant women is based on net, rather than gross, income, it is fair to assume that virtually all of these births would be eligible for Medicaid payment in whole or part. Even births to undocumented women would be eligible for coverage, at least with respect to those costs that are attributable to active labor.

16. Congressional Budget Office, *Factors Contributing to the Growth of the Medicaid Program* (Washington, D.C., May 1992), p. 18.

17. For example, the Alan Guttmacher Institute, in *Blessed Events and the Bottom Line* (Washington, D.C., 1987), estimated that 17 percent of all births in the United States were Medicaid financed. Given the fact that not all Medicaid-eligible women enroll in the program, it is probably safe to assume that, prior to the expansions, between 20 and 25 percent of all births in the United States were eligible for payment in whole or in part.

18. Conversation with Russell Toal, Director, Georgia Medicaid Agency, June 2, 1992.

19. See, U.S. General Accounting Office, *Prenatal Care: Early Success in Enrolling Women Made Eligible by Medicaid Expansions* (GAO/PEMD-91-10, February 1991).

20. See H. Rep. No. 101-M to Accompany H.R. 2924, as incorporated into H.R. 3299, the Omnibus Budget Reconciliation Act of 1989. By July 1989, 44 states and the District of Columbia covered all poor pregnant women and infants with family incomes below 100 percent of the federal poverty level. Twenty-one states covered all poor children under age 5, and 14 covered poor children up to age 8. H. Rep. No. 101-M at p.52.

21. This delay in coverage may also mean that, rather than being cost-reducing, Medicaid coverage may initially add to program costs. To the extent that the Medicaid reforms succeed in enrolling additional numbers of women in poor health well into their pregnancies, the immediate result may be increased numbers of relatively expensive, high risk births and an increased incidence of infant mortality among the Medicaid population. Obviously this in no way negates the importance of the reforms; indeed, if anything, it strengthens their importance, because furnishing medical care to these women and children is particularly important. But this potential result certainly must be taken into account in determining if the Medicaid reforms have in fact been associated with a reduction in infant mortality or cost-savings.

22. Physician Payment Review Commission, *Annual Report to Congress, 1992* (Washington, D.C.) pp. 141–83.

23. See, e.g., Physician Payment Review Commission, *Physician Payment Under Medicaid*, No. 91-4 (Washington, D.C., 1991); Physician Payment Review Commission, *Annual Report to Congress, 1992* (Washington, D.C.); Lewis, I., *Increasing Provider Participation* (Washington, D.C.: National Governors Association, 1988); U.S. General Accounting Office, *Prenatal Care: Medicaid Recipients and Uninsured Women Obtain Insufficient Care* HRD-87-137 (Washington, D.C., September, 1987).

24. Physicians Payment Review Commission, *Annual Report to Congress, 1992* (Washington, D.C.); Fossett, J. "Medicaid in the Inner City: The Case of Maternity Care in Chicago," *Milbank Quarterly* 68:1 (1990), pp. 111–141.

25. Buescher, P., Roth, M., Williams, D., and Goforth, C., "An Evaluation of the Impact of Maternity Care Coordination on Medicaid Birth Outcomes in North Carolina," *AJPH* 81:12 (December, 1991), pp. 1625–1629; Buescher, P., and Ward, N., "A Comparison of Low Birthweight Among Medicaid Patients of Public Health Departments and Other Providers of Prenatal Care in North Carolina and Kentucky," *Public Health Reports* 107:1 (January–February, 1992), pp. 54–59.

26. American Academy of Pediatrics, *Health Care Financing Newsletter*, 1992.

27. To be eligible for Medicaid, persons must be residents of the state in which they apply for benefits. Normally Medicaid defines residency as living in a particular place with an intent to permanently reside there. However, in the case of migrant families, the program recognizes residency even if a person or family is only temporarily in a state for job-related reasons.

28. See, Rosenbaum, S., and Liu, J., *Medicaid and Migrant Farmworker Families: Analysis of Barriers and Recommendations for Change* (Washington, D.C.: National Association of Community Health Centers) July 1991.

29. 42 U.S.C. §§1396a(a)(10)(B) and 1396d (1980).

30. This option was provided as a result of the regulatory creation in 1967 of the AFDC "unborn child" program. The Department of Health, Education, and Welfare, following adoption of this expanded cash assistance option, amended its policies regarding Medicaid coverage of financially needy children under age 21 to include "unborn" children.

31. By 1983, less than half of all states covered all financially needy children, including unborn children. See H. Rep. No. 98–442 to Accompany H.R. 4136, the Deficit Reduction Amendments of 1983.

32. See, e.g., Davis, K., and Schoen, C., *Health and the War on Poverty* (Washington, D.C.: Brookings Press, 1977). It is perhaps also worth noting that in commenting on the significant decline in infant mortality for 1990, as measured by provisional 1990 statistics, Secretary of Health and Human Services, Dr. Louis Sullivan, attributed at least a portion of the reduction to the expanded Medicaid benefits and the greater ambulatory and inpatient care access they produced.

33. See, e.g., Korenbrot, C.C., *Risk Reduction in Pregnancies of Low Income Women; Comprehensive Prenatal Care Through the OB Access Project* (University of California at San Francisco: Center for Reproductive Health, Institute for Health Policy Studies, 1984); Buescher, P.A., and Ward, N.I., "A Comparison of Low Birthweight Among Medicaid Patients of Public Health Departments and Other Providers of Prenatal Care in North Carolina and Kentucky," *Public Health Reports* 107:54–59 (1992); Buescher, P.A., et al., "A comparison of Women in and out of a Prematurity Prevention Project in a North Carolina Perinatal Care Region," *American Journal of Public Health* 78:264–267 (1988); Utah Health Department, "Preliminary Evaluation of the Impact of Medicaid Expansions on Utah's Infant Mortality Rate" (Salt Lake City, Ut., 1991) (unpublished).

34. While PE does not entitle women to payment for inpatient care, the cost of such care can be covered retroactively, once eligibility is determined.

35. 42 U.S.C. §1396a(a)(4) (1992). In many OE settings the out-stationed worker is a staff or contract employee of the welfare agency. In these cases, the full eligibility determination process can be completed on-site.

36. The law requires that "initial" eligibility determinations take place at the OE site. In implementing OE, the Health Care Financing Administration has defined "initial" determinations to include completion of applications, gathering of documentation, and applicant interviews, if required. Left to the "final" process (which can take place at the OE site if a welfare agency employee is used) is verification of documentation and final eligibility determination.

37. See, Institute of Medicine, *Prenatal Care: Reaching Mothers, Reaching Infants* (Washington, D.C.: National Academy Press, 1988), pp. 72–76, and studies cited therein; Shuptrine, S., and Grant, V., *The Relationship of the Reasons for Denial of AFDC/Medicaid Benefits to the Uninsured in the United States* (Columbia, S.C., 1988).

38. It is interesting to note that except for documentation of lawful U.S. status, there are no statutory or regulatory definitions regarding what is acceptable verification of eligibility. Federal law does prohibit the states from requiring certain forms of residency verification (i.e., proof of an address) in the case of applicants who are homeless. But the type of documentation that is acceptable to show age or pregnancy status appears to be left to the states.

39. This does not mean, however, that eligibility lasts for a year. Any change in an enrollee's status must be reported and eligibility must be redetermined at that point.

40. U.S. General Accounting Office, *Prenatal Care: Early Success in Enrolling Women Made Eligible by Medicaid Expansions* (Washington, D.C.: GAO/PEMD 91–10, February 1991). Whether temporary coverage provided through PE actually has increased women's access to early care is not known. Many women already may be receiving care from the providers who perform the PE determination, so that finding a source of care is not the issue. In assessing the value of PE, however, it is extremely important to measure not only its impact on finding an entry point in to care but also its impact on the ability of prenatal providers to secure specialized out-patient services (e.g., referrals to medical specialists for high risk women, special laboratory tests or medications) that are not provided on-site.

41. The Alameda Health Consortium, a consortium of health centers and community clinics located in Alameda County, California, reports high success in retaining coverage for patients by assisting in both the initial enrollment and eligibility redetermination process. See, generally, Silber, R., and Hughes, D., "Out-stationed Enrollment for Pregnant Women and Children" (Oakland, CA: Alameda Health Consortium, 1990).

42. Congressional Budget Office, *Factors Contributing to the Growth of the Medicaid Program* (Washington, D.C., May 1992) p. 18.

43. Rosenbaum, S., and Rivera, L., *An Evaluation of Out-stationed Enrollment Implementation at Community and Migrant Health Centers* (Washington, D.C.: Children's Defense Fund, March 1992).

44. As with so much of Medicaid today, while there is HCFA guidance on OE, there are no formally issued rules. However, on many aspects of the OE program, the HCFA guidance is quite clear.

45. This position is reinforced by the Medicaid Moratorium Amendments of 1991, which permit provider donations for certain types of OE programs and which thus at least implicitly provide that in the absence of donations, responsibility for payment rests with the states. It is not clear that the real concern is with the cost of the OE process itself, however. A fulltime OE worker at a clinic probably costs about $30,000 annually, half of which is borne by the federal government as an administration cost. It may be that not aggressively implementing OE is in fact more a mechanism for controlling program caseload size in particularly hard-pressed states.

46. Medicaid eligibility for aged, blind, and disabled persons is based on the financial criteria used for determining eligibility for Supplemental Security Income (SSI) benefits. Income eligibility is set at approximately 85 percent of the federal poverty level, while allowable asset levels are $2,000 for an individual and $3,000 for a couple.

47. The adverse impact of high out-of-pocket burdens on low-income Medicare beneficiaries has been well documented. See, Rowland, D., "Fewer Resources, Greater Burdens: Medical Care Coverage for Low Income Elderly People" in U.S. Bipartisan Commission on Health Care, *A Call for Action* (Washington, D.C., 1990) Vol. III.

48. It should be noted, however, that the QMB protections assure payment only of Part B premium costs in the case of QMBs with incomes over the federal poverty level.

49. Families USA, *Still a Government Secret* (Washington, D.C., 1992). This report was predated by a 1991 report, also issued by Families USA, which first documented the low rate of enrollment in the QMB program.

50. The report does not indicate what percentage of low-income disabled Medicare beneficiaries are not enrolled in the QMB program.

51. Mandatory Medicaid payment of part B premiums and cost-sharing for dually enrolled Medicare beneficiaries were added to the statute after the QMB program for non-dually enrolled persons was adopted.

52. It is difficult to imagine that it would be higher. Elderly persons not receiving SSI probably would apply for Medicaid only to pay for high-cost, uncovered Medicare services such as long-term care.

53. The American Public Welfare Association, for example, in 1991 recommended amending Medicaid to permit QMB enrollment at Social Security offices.

54. For example, about 15 percent of all poor children do have some form of third-party coverage. Yet the governors have supported extending Medicaid benefits to all poor children in recognition of the inadequacy of most third-party coverage for the poor.

55. For example, FHQCs are entitled to payment for 100 percent of the reasonable cost of their covered services. Since Medicare only pays 80 percent of the reasonable cost, apparently at least partial Medicaid payment would always be due. Yet HCFA has indicated that states' obligation to cover these copayments is unclear. In the case of FQHC services, there would be no state responsibility to pay the Medicare Part B deductible for QMBs, however. In 1990, Congress waived application of the deductible in the case of Part B FQHC services. This was done because low-income elderly health center patients, like other CHC

patients, are eligible for the income-adjusted fees that community health centers are required to charge. Rather than leaving health centers with high uncovered costs to be borne by their Public Health Service grants or shifting responsibility for the costs to state Medicaid programs, Congress determined that Medicare should bear the cost.

56. 42 U.S.C. §1396d(a) (1992). Virtually all types of medical and remedial care and services for which federal financial participation is available under the statute are listed in this section of the law.

57. Preliminary guidance from the agency, however, indicates that HCFA does indeed view the amendments as having fundamentally altered the pediatric component of Medicaid and eliminated the "fire wall" between EPSDT and the rest of pediatric Medicaid coverage policy. Indeed, HCFA's response to the program has thus far been notable for the strong position it has taken regarding the states' obligation to extend comprehensive medical care to children on an as-needed basis, regardless of whether the treatment is needed for a new condition or one whose existence was known prior to the EPSDT screen.

58. See, Rosenbaum, S., and Johnson, K., "Providing Health Care for Low Income Children: Reconciling Child Health Goals with Child Health Financing Realities," *Milbank Quarterly* 64:3, 442–478 (1986).

59. It is interesting to note that the original proposed rules required the states to pay for all medically necessary treatment children needed, even if not otherwise covered in their state plans for adults. After resistance from the states, the Nixon Administration scaled back the requirement to vision, dental, and hearing care only. The states were given the option to pay for all care needed to treat conditions found during a screen.

60. The federal government's delay resulted in litigation against the Department of Health, Education, and Welfare in 1970. *NWRO v. Weinberger*, No. 70–1276 (D.D.C., 1970).

61. Section 403, P.L. 92–603, The Social Security Amendments of 1972.

62. This is ironic given the current involvement by Medicaid agencies in the creation of managed care systems that provide for care as well as pay for it. In 1972, however, this notion seemed far more radical.

63. *Stanton v. Bond*, 504 F.2d 1246 (7th Cir., 1974). The plaintiffs in *Bond* challenged the state's virtual failure to make the new benefits available. In its ruling in plaintiffs' favor, the United States Court of Appeals articulated the program's overarching preventive health care standard on which all subsequent EPSDT litigation was based.

64. See, e.g., *Harris v. Candon*, No. 77–424 (N.D. Vt., 1978).

65 See, e.g., *Mitchell v. Johnston*, 701 F.2d 337 (5th Cir., 1983); *PWRO v. Schapp*, 602 F.2d 1134 (3rd Cir., 1979); *Brooks v. Smith* (Me. Supreme Judicial Court, 1976).

66. Section 2164, P.L. 97–35, Omnibus Budget Reconciliation Act of 1981.

67. 42 U.S.C. §1396a(a)(43).

68. It is worth noting that while HCFA has developed a universal provider claims form for Medicaid agencies, only after numerous comments did the agency add a field to the form allowing providers to report the encounter as an EPSDT screen. Thus, HCFA helped perpetuate a bifurcated provider claims system for pediatric health care, thereby further confusing the matter.

69. St. Peter, R., Newacheck, P., and Halfon, N., "Access to Care for Poor Children: Separate and Unequal?" *JAMA* 267:20, pp. 2760–2764 (May 27, 1992); Rosenbach, M., *Insurance Coverage and Ambulatory Medical Care of Low Income Children, 1980* (Series C, Analytical Report #1) (Washington, D.C., 1985).

70. This is a common problem. See, Liu, J., and Rosenbaum, S., *Medicaid and Childhood Immunizations* (Washington, D.C.: Children's Defense Fund, 1992).

71. The failure to cover mental health and developmental disability–related services became more pressing with passage in 1986 of Part H of the Individuals with Disabilities Education Act (IDEA). The Part H program authorizes comprehensive early intervention services for infants and toddlers with, or at risk for, developmental disabilities and delays. While Part H funds case finding, treatment plan development, evaluation, and case management, it provides no funds for treatment. Like the special education program for handicapped children, early intervention services are a mix of therapeutic, rehabilitation, and child development services to help disabled infants and toddlers overcome or minimize actual or potential disabilities. There was great concern with passage of the Act that the poorest Part H–eligible, disabled infants and toddlers (about 7 percent of all poor children under age 3) would be identified and assessed but that there would be no funds for their care. As a result, Part H was crafted to assume that Medicaid will pay for the therapeutic care a Medicaid-enrolled baby needs. Moreover, in 1988 Medicaid was amended, as part of the Medicare Catastrophic Coverage Act, to require state payment for covered care and services for disabled infants and toddlers. The 1989 EPSDT amendments thus were an attempt to assure that in all states, such services would be covered. See, Orloff, T., Rivera, L., Harris, P., and Rosenbaum, S., *Medicaid and Early Intervention Under Part H of the Individuals With Disabilities Act* (Washington, D.C.: Children's Defense Fund, 1992).

72. The Medicare FFHC program was created by rule in 1966 and provided for cost-based reimbursement for the OEO neighborhood health centers. In 1990, after the FQHC program was added to the Medicaid statute, Congress codified the FFHC program as a permanent part B benefit, also known as federally qualified health centers.

73. As of January 1992, data from the Public Health Service Bureau of Health Care Delivery Assistance show that of 130 applications for look-alike certification received to date, 73 had been approved. Of these, 22 involved public entities and 51 involved private entities.

74. Of the 73 FQHCs approved as of January 1992, only 14 were approved without waivers. Fifteen (all but three of which were public) had received waivers of the 24-hour coverage requirement. Three had received waivers of the fee schedule. One had received waivers of the inpatient continuity requirement. Forty-one had received waivers of the requirement that at least 51 percent of the health center's governing board be comprised of users of the center.

75. There is no way of knowing for sure how many of these entities there are. At the time of enactment, the National Association of Community Health Centers estimated that there were between 300 and 500 entities that met all of the criteria of the community health centers program but received no federal funds. This number, however, does not take into account existing entities that modify their program content and governance structure to meet the federal health center criteria.

76. FQHC services specifically include the services of physicians and mid-level practitioners and services and supplies incident to their services, as well as services of certain psychologists and social workers. 42 U.S.C. §1395x(aa) (1992). In the case of Medicare, FQHC services also include coverage for preventive services. As noted above, the Medicare FQHC benefit is available on a first-dollar basis without payment of a deductible. 42 U.S.C. §§1395l(a) and (b) (1992).

77. 42 U.S.C. §1396a(a)(13)(E).

78. See, generally, Physician Payment Review Commission, *Physician Payment Under Medicaid* No. 91–4 (Washington, D.C., 1991).

79. Ibid.

80. Davis, K., and Schoen, C., *Health and the War on Poverty* (Washington, D.C.: Brookings Press, 1977); Sardell, A., *The U.S. Social Experiment* (University of Pittsburgh Press, 1990). While many of the health center studies are quite old, more recent studies of comprehensive health care programs exhibiting the attributes of health centers have reached the same conclusion—namely, that programs with certain health care characteristics achieve good health outcomes for children.

81. Falik, M., Lewis-Idema, D., and Norton, J., *Implementation Status of Federally Qualified Health Center Reimbursements, as of September, 1991* (Washington, D.C.: National Association of Community Health Centers, 1991).

82. See footnote 71, *supra*.

•

4

Medicaid Payment Policy and the Boren Amendment

GERARD ANDERSON AND WILLIAM SCANLON

INTRODUCTION

The Boren Amendment sets a federal standard for determining the reasonableness of payment rates to hospitals and nursing homes in the Medicaid program. Originally enacted in 1980 to affirm the states' prerogative to pursue cost containment in setting nursing home payment rates, and amended a year later to encourage similar action regarding hospitals, it has been used repeatedly in recent years as the basis for lawsuits challenging some states' payment rates to both hospitals and nursing homes. While the payment rates of Medicaid programs have frequently been affirmed by courts, there is increasing concern that the vague and imprecise language of the Boren Amendment makes it difficult for the states to defend policies that fall within the range of their discretion.

Recent court decisions have created a concern among the states that the courts may improperly limit their discretion to set payment rates as the courts become increasingly involved in specifics of payment methodology. The court decisions raise the fundamental issues of what is an appropriate payment rate and who should certify that the payment rate is appropriate. In addition, recent decisions have questioned not only the states "substantive" compliance but "procedural" compliance as well. These decisions create the potential that the states will have to undertake extensive, detailed analyses to defend their rates. Decisions that have gone against the states raise the additional issue of who should allocate resources, since higher rates paid to institutional providers either as a direct result of a court decision or as a guard against possible future adverse decisions may divert resources from expansions in coverage or eligibility that state and federal policymakers may find preferable.

HISTORY OF THE BOREN AMENDMENT

The Boren Amendment was adopted in two stages. Incorporated in the Omnibus Reconciliation Act of 1980, the Amendment established a criterion for payment to skilled nursing facilities (SNFs) and intermediate case facilities (ICFs). The Omnibus Budget Reconciliation Act of 1981 modified the Amendment's language to include hospitals. The final language specified that:

> A state plan for medical assistance must provide for payment... of the *hospital,* SNF and ICF services provided under the plan through the use of rates (determined in accordance with methods and standards developed by the State *and which, in the case of hospitals, take into account the situation of hospitals which serve a disproportionate number of low income patients with special needs...* which the state finds and makes assurances satisfactory to the Secretary, are reasonable and adequate to meet the costs that must be incurred by efficiently and economically operated facilities to provide care and services in conformity with applicable State and Federal laws, regulations, and quality and safety standards *and to assure that individuals eligible for medical assistance have reasonable access (taking into account geographic location and reasonable travel time) to inpatient hospital services of adequate quality.* (The 1981 changes which are applicable only to hospitals are in italics.)

Although the Boren Amendment uses essentially the same language for nursing homes and hospitals, the legislative history, the role of Medicaid in determining the financial status of nursing homes or hospitals, and judicial experience differ considerably for those institutions. With respect to nursing homes, it is generally agreed that the Boren Amendment was intended primarily to strengthen existing legislation in which Congress already had given the states discretion in setting payment rates. Prior to 1972, there were no federal requirements for SNF payment, which at the time was the only Medicaid-covered nursing home service. As part of the 1972 Amendments to the Social Security Act (P.L. 92–603), which made a large number of program changes (including extending Medicaid coverage to ICFs), Congress enacted Section 249, requiring that payments to SNFs and ICFs be on a reasonable cost–related basis using methods acceptable to the Secretary of Health, Education, and Welfare, now Health and Human Services (HHS). The states were free to adopt Medicare's principles of retrospective reasonable cost reimbursement or to develop other methods, which had to be approved by the Secretary. The motivation for the 1972 change, as expressed in the Committee Report, was to bring payment rates into what Congress perceived as a more acceptable range. Congress had heard testimony that revealed that payments to some SNFs and ICFs were too high and to others too insufficient to cover the cost of minimum quality care.

The impetus for the Boren Amendment in 1980 for nursing homes was a concern that the approval process established by the Health Care Financing Administration (HCFA) and court decisions in lawsuits challenging HCFA's and the states' compliance with Section 249 were forcing the states to adopt Medicare's methods. The Senate Finance Committee in its Report on the Boren Amendment indicated that this was not the original intent of Section 249.

> The Committee continues to believe that States should have flexibility in developing methods of payment for their Medicaid programs and that application of the reasonable cost reimbursement principles of the Medicare program for long-term care facility services is not entirely satisfactory.

While the states were given latitude to promote cost containment, the Committee was clearly concerned that cost containment not be pursued at beneficiaries' expense. It therefore stated that the Boren Amendment was "not intended to encourage arbitrary reductions in payment that would adversely affect the quality of care."

In 1981, Congress used the language of the Boren Amendment with some modifications and applied it to hospitals. Its adoption resulted from concerns about the rapid increase in Medicaid expenditures (an average annual rate of 16 percent during the 1970s) and the Reagan Administration's interest in reducing Medicaid spending. From Medicaid's inception in 1966, the states had been required to use Medicare's retrospective cost reimbursement methods to pay hospitals. Exceptions were allowed only if a state obtained an HCFA waiver.

Giving the states greater flexibility to develop their own hospital payment system was seen as contributing to the control of health care costs, since cost-based reimbursement methods were viewed by the Senate Finance Committee to be "inherently inflationary and contain no incentives for efficient performance." While cost containment may have been the primary goal, the responsible congressional committees expressed concern that arbitrary and unduly low rates could compromise either access or quality of care. They consequently made consideration of these impacts part of the Amendment and gave final authority to approve rates to the Secretary of HHS.

In enacting the Boren Amendment, Congress also made clear its intention to maintain federal oversight to insure the adequacy of rates while granting the states some discretion. Experience with nursing home payment prior to 1972 and physician payment throughout the program's history had produced some unsatisfactory results. Without federal oversight of rates, some states set them well below those of other payers and created problems of access and/or quality of care for Medicaid eligibles (1). Congress explicitly recognized this problem in the Committee Reports and reaffirmed its desire that the rates paid to institutional providers meet some standard of adequacy in the Omnibus Reconciliation Act of 1990 (P.L. 101–508), which further modified the Boren Amendment to require that the cost of implementing the 1987 nursing home quality reforms be taken into account.

The states have made considerable use of the flexibility granted by the Boren Amendment. As of 1989, 42 states had adopted some form of prospective payment for hospitals, and more states have developed prospective payment systems for nursing homes. As the states have developed payment rates that paid some nursing homes and hospitals less than their full costs, the providers have sued, citing the language in the Boren Amendment that requires states to pay rates that are "reasonable and adequate to meet the costs which must be incurred by efficiently and economically operated facilities." The absence of clear and precise definitions for efficient and economic providers or for what costs must be incurred in either the statute or the implementing regulations has been responsible for most of the litigation.

TRENDS IN BOREN AMENDMENT LITIGATION

The court cases challenging Medicaid payment rates have involved a range of procedural and substantive issues (2). While there are some trends emerging from the cases, most policy issues have not been litigated sufficiently to arrive at any clear judicial standard.

One trend relates to the importance of adhering to procedures that the Boren Amendment requires for validating state plan amendments. The 1983 regulations that accompany the Boren Amendment specify that the states are required to make assurances to the Secretary of HHS that the state plan meets the requirements of the statute. Carefully adhering to congressional instructions contained in the Committee Reports, HCFA declined to require explicit definitions of efficiently and economically operated providers, to define a methodology for reviewing these assurances, to require that the states submit written findings to support their assurances, or, in the case of hospitals, to set minimum standards for payment to disproportionate share hospitals. In the early cases, the courts presumed that if HCFA had approved a state plan, then the state must have followed the necessary regulatory procedures.

A 1989 federal appellate court decision (*AMISUB v. State of Colorado Department of Social Services*), which set out specific requirements for the findings process, represented a major departure from that line of reasoning. The court ruled that state Medicaid agencies are required:

> at a minimum, to make 'findings' which identify and determine (1) efficiently and economically operated hospitals; (2) the costs that must be incurred by such hospitals; and, (3) payment rates which are reasonable and adequate to meet the reasonable costs of the State's efficiently and economically operated hospitals.

These requirements were specified in a case where the violation of the Boren Amendment seems clear. Colorado had imposed ceilings on costs to be recognized for rate setting and then multiplied all remaining costs by 54 percent in order to stay within a budget target. Subsequent courts have not focussed on the circumstances of *AMISUB*. Instead, they have relied on the three-factor test to invalidate state plan amendments that failed to adhere to these procedures and required that they occur before payment method changes are implemented. A recent decision involving nursing homes in Illinois was based solely on the state's judged failure to meet the procedural requirements. That failure made the substance of the system irrelevant in the eyes of the court.

These procedural standards have important substantive implications. The states are required to undertake analyses to define and measure provider efficiency and then to adopt findings comparing the costs of efficient hospitals with the state payment rates. Unfortunately, there are no commonly accepted definitions of these terms or precise ways to measure efficiency or economy, and there is a disagreement with respect to how costs should be measured. For example, the economists' definition of efficiency, producing a product at the lowest possible cost, and the common definition of economical, utilitarian, or not extravagant, are difficult to make operational. Even if some consensus on the meanings of these critical tasks could be achieved, the burden of testing compliance for individual providers would be considerable. Many states have hundreds of hospitals and nursing homes participating in Medicaid. Subjecting their operations, which differ widely in structure and process, to a detailed analysis and evaluation to measure operational efficiency and economy would be a huge undertaking.

These difficulties may deter the states from ever adopting innovative payment methods that strongly promote efficiency or economy since they may be unable to unambiguously demonstrate the legitimacy of such methods. The states may be left in the bind of having to pay more than is truly required by the Boren Amendment simply to establish beyond any doubt that the costs of efficient and economical providers have been paid.

A second trend relates to the degree of discretion that the courts will grant to the states in the design of their payment systems. In early cases, the courts ruled solely on whether the states had acted in an arbitrary and capricious manner. In later cases, courts have closely scrutinized the specific components of a payment system, with judges becoming increasingly willing to make decisions that previously had been left to the state administration. The *AMISUB* court explicitly held that the federal courts do not owe state agencies the same deference they owe federal agencies and so held that compliance with the Boren Amendment "is an issue of law subject to *de novo* review in federal court."

This standard of review explicitly invites courts to substitute their judgment for that of the states in determining the appropriate payment rate. Increasingly, the courts have been willing to review the specifics of rate setting methodologies as they have seen other courts review such details. It is also possible that some of the recent decisions are reacting to more aggressive state efforts to reduce payments. Early cases often involved relatively modest efforts at cost containment—a short-term rate freeze or inflation adjustments slightly below the growth in costs. In contrast, some recent cases have challenged large, across-the-board reductions to meet a specific budget target or the cumulative results of many years of cost-containment activities.

While these recent court decisions may have reflected congressional intent and corrected certain abuses, they raise concerns on two fronts. First, the perspective on cost containment in health care has shifted since the enactment of the Boren Amendment. Evidence of this shift is exemplified in the adoption of the Medicare Prospective Payment System (PPS) for hospitals. PPS rates created strong financial incentives for hospitals to deliver a more economical product and to become more efficient in its delivery. When Medicaid programs try to emulate PPS rates or apply PPS principles, gaps between rates and costs are likely to occur. It is therefore possible that Medicare rates will be declared inappropriate for Medicaid since Medicare no longer uses costs as its standard to set rates. Indeed, two nursing home cases (Indiana and New York) have invalidated payment systems that are structurally very similar to PPS.

The second concern stems from some cases where state payment systems may have violated the Boren standard and the courts have singled out isolated components of the system for criticism. The concern is that these critiques will become a precedent for future decisions that might invalidate a system because of a specific component rather than because of how the total rate compared to total cost. To do so would be counter to an early decision in a New York case, which seemed to establish a reasonable method of reviewing a total system. This decision affirmed the state's system despite an apparent deficiency in the capital payment because other features were likely to compensate and result in adequate rates. Besides creating the risk of inappropriately striking down a system because of an individual component, focusing judicial review on individual components substantially increases the analysis states may have to undertake to defend their choices.

The scenario envisioned by the dissenting Justices in the U.S. Supreme Court's *Wilder* decision may become a reality: "providers. . .will inevitably seek the substitution of a rate system preferred by the provider for the rate system chosen by the State." If the court decides in favor of the provider, then the states will be required "to adopt reimbursement rate systems different from those Congress expressly required them to adopt...." The end result may not be a system that emerges from a coherent policy development process. Instead, it is likely to be specifically geared toward meeting the needs of the plaintiff providers and responding to the mandate of the court.

A related implication is that the court cases will result in significant increase in Medicaid program expenditures in addition to outlays for legal costs. For instance, as a result of the *Temple* decision, Pennsylvania estimates that its state-wide Medicaid outlays were increased by 15 percent, and in Washington state, hospital payment rates were ordered to be increased by 9 percent. In Virginia, 91 hospitals negotiated a settlement after *Wilder*, under which they will receive rate increases totaling $120 million over four years. In addition to these identifiable costs, Medicaid outlays are higher because state officials may choose to forego payment system changes that would promote greater efficiency or economy out of fear of the legal challenge that will result. While potentially impossible to measure, these latter increases may dwarf those emanating directly from the lawsuits or well-documented negotiations.

OPTIONS FOR REFORM OF THE BOREN AMENDMENT

The need for reform of the Boren Amendment is obvious. The primary reason is that the uncertainty created by the Boren Amendment is potentially preventing the states from controlling rates to institutional providers in ways that compromise neither access nor quality. It is also forcing many to defend rates that may be fully compliant with the Boren Amendment. The cost and the cause of such unnecessary actions were noted in a decision in a Washington state hospital case: "The failure of Congress or the Secretary of Health and Human Services to define these critical terms has caused the States to expend millions of dollars in attempting to comply with these amorphous terms."

A number of alternatives to the current law are described in the following paragraphs. The alternatives include precisely defining the terms of the Boren Amendment; restricting court review; and requiring that Medicaid become the lowest cost payer, removing all references to cost, removing all discretion from the states, or accepting all payer rates. In considering proposed options, the balance between the budgetary concerns of the states, access to and quality of hospital and nursing home services, equitable treatment of providers and other payers, and the competing demands of other service needs to be weighed carefully.

In reviewing the options, it is important to consider the differences in the structure of the hospital and nursing home industries and the role that Medicaid plays for each provider. Hospitals produce a large number of distinct products for which timely access is critical to patients' well being. They have been constrained little by market or regulatory forces to control either their capacity or their costs—resulting in the perception that there is considerable excess in both. Finally, Medicaid is a relatively small purchaser of care, representing 10 percent of revenues in the average hospital (while there is a much higher concentration in a few hospitals, many serve almost no Medicaid patients).

Nursing homes are almost totally opposite. They produce a relatively homogenous product for which timely access is not an issue, as hospital stays and home care are frequently short- and intermediate-term substitutes.

They have been constrained considerably by both market and regulatory forces. Their principal customers are persons paying out of pocket and Medicaid. Private patients are presumably somewhat competent consumers able and willing to shop among homes for the best product consistent with the price. Since need for nursing home care is not immediate, as is often the case with hospital care, consumers have time to make an informed choice. Medicaid programs have also been aggressive consumers since nursing home spending involves more than a third of the program's budget in most states. The state's limits on bed construction, their principal tool in controlling spending, are seen as resulting in excess demand, rather than excess capacity, in a large number of areas. Medicaid's large share of patients, 60 to 65 percent in most states, means that homes have little choice but to participate and serve the program's patients. The program's market share and use of payment methods to encourage cost containment, combined with private patients' sensitivity to price, are seen as reducing, but not eliminating, the extent of inefficiency relative to hospitals.

These differences mean that options that may be very attractive for hospitals may be much less so, or even undesirable, to implement for nursing homes. This should not be a great concern. There appears to be little or anything to gain from requiring that the same solution be applied to both provider types. Indeed, considering each industry separately, at least at the outset, may be the more desirable approach.

Precisely Define Terms in the Boren Amendment

Precise definition of the key terms in the Boren Amendment, either by HCFA through regulation or by Congress through legislation, could resolve much of the uncertainty. The advantage of this approach would be to limit the scope of issues open for judicial review. The language in the greatest need of clarification is the phrase "costs that must be incurred by the efficiently and economically operated facilities." It may be helpful, but likely not sufficient to resolve much of the uncertainty, if Congress or HCFA provided a more detailed conceptual definition of these terms. What is really needed is guidance on how states can determine these costs empirically with a reasonable amount of administrative resources. The Propspective Payment Assessment Commission (ProPAC) has suggested that HCFA clarify the language in the Boren Amendment, and so far HCFA has declined, citing the original legislative language that gave tremendous flexibility to the states (3).

Another approach would be for Congress to be more precise about the procedural steps the states and HCFA must take in adopting, supporting, and reviewing payment rates (eliminating the need for judicial imposition of the *AMISUB* standards). This would not make the substantive issues any less contentious, but it would assist in their being resolved at the administrative level without excessive judicial intervention.

Restrict Court Review

Judicial review of Medicaid rates for institutional care could be restricted or eliminated. The Medicare PPS is not subject to judicial review of its basic methodology. A similar provision could be introduced for the Medicaid program. The advantage is that it would reduce the amount of litigation. However, it would raise the issue of who will monitor state actions. It may be necessary for Congress or the Secretary of HHS to designate that HCFA have primary responsibility to determine compliance with the Boren Amendment. While it might subject the states to closer scrutiny than at present, it would make the reviews more consistent by concentrating them in a single entity with considerable technical expertise. Hospitals, nursing homes, and beneficiaries, however, might be concerned that the federal government's financial support of Medicaid would give it a biased perspective.

Medicaid as Lowest Cost Payer

Rather than try to define what is the cost of an efficient provider, Medicaid could be permitted to examine a provider's agreements with other insurers and allow Medicaid to match the best deal the provider gave to any other insurer. This is similar to the approach Congress adopted in 1990 with respect to payment for drugs in the Medicaid program. Under this provision, Medicaid pays the rate that a drug company gives to its best customers.

The major advantage of this approach is that it would set an objective standard that is relatively easy to administer, and it would assure the Medicaid program the lowest rate. This approach has proved disastrous with respect to drugs since no single purchaser has the market power to resist price increases promulgated by drug manufacturers. The approach might have more positive results with hospitals, since there is more negotiation over hospital rates. In most states, however, Medicaid already pays the lowest rate to hospitals. For nursing homes this option may not be feasible or effective since Medicaid and self-pay patients are essentially the only two payers, and again Medicaid is usually the lowest payer already.

Substitute Access and Quality Standards for Cost in the Language of the Boren Amendment

Instead of cost, the emphasis could be given to providing access and quality health care to Medicaid recipients. For example, the language could be revised to require that the states set payment rates that assure reasonable access to quality care. A second approach would require the states to pay rates sufficient to attract enough licensed providers to meet each state's projection of need. In other words, pay what is necessary to get Medicaid recipients adequate care.

Empirical standards for access and quality would have to be clearly defined. It would be essential to tailor the standards to specific market conditions so that Medicaid is not forced to support grossly inefficient providers to assure access in sparsely populated areas.

Establish a Uniform Prospective Payment System for the Medicaid Program

To ensure that states are paying reasonable rates, Congress could mandate that Medicaid programs use a uniform methodology. The disadvantage of this approach is that it eliminates states' discretion and would probably result in higher payments in many states. This contradicts the notion inherent in the basic design of Medicaid that the program is a joint state/federal undertaking. The advantage of this approach would be the elimination of the need for HCFA oversight of state plans. It probably would not benefit Medicaid recipients by improving either access or quality of care for hospital and nursing home care.

Selective Contracting Based on Competitive Bidding

A few states, notably California, have moved toward a competitive approach by selectively contracting with a limited number of hospitals based on competitive bids. The consensual nature of the resulting reimbursement rate removes these cases from the likelihood of a Boren Amendment dispute. However, it requires Medicaid waivers since it restricts access to certain hospitals. In addition, selective contracting may be difficult to implement in more sparsely populated states where there may be a much thinner hospital market, and such contracting would not be feasible in the nursing home market where Medicaid is such a dominant purchaser.

Accepting All-Payer Rates

Since 1970, a number of states have instituted all-payer rate setting systems. An all-payer system is one that imposes a centralized rate-setting methodology to control the amount hospitals or nursing homes can charge any patient, whether privately or publicly insured, or whether insured at all. In general, these programs have shown considerable success in controlling the rate of increase in hospital costs when they adopt a mandatory, binding methodology. Some of these state systems have equalized payment rates across payers; others have institutionalized existing payment differentials; and still others have attempted to reduce the differential over time. Experience with all-payer rate setting for nursing homes (Minnesota and North Dakota) is more limited and less well documented because comparable data by state are not routinely collected.

If all-payer rates were deemed in compliance with Medicaid standards, it would subsume disputes over Medicaid reimbursement since they would be part of disputes over their entire rate structure. The advantage of this approach is that it would maintain state flexibility in design of the system. However, adopting all-payer rate regulation at the state level is a highly politicized decision, extending well beyond Medicaid, especially with regard to hospitals, and is not likely to be undertaken quickly on a widespread basis.

Assessment of the Options

Assessment of how implementation of any of these options will affect Medicaid cost or access to and quality of care for Medicaid beneficiaries is not a simple exercise. Each of the options discussed are generic, requiring choice about numerous details before they can be considered to be fully specified. Given the states' concerns that litigation under the Boren Amendment hinders their efforts at cost containment and providers' concerns over inadequate payment rates, it is unclear what direction Congress will take. Likewise, how the states would respond to any of these proposals is unclear, as is the response of the hospital and nursing home industries. For hospitals, responses may be more muted since participation in the Medicare and Medicaid program is bundled together. It is unlikely that any hospital would want to stop participating in the Medicare program. For almost all nursing homes, there may not be an option either since the Medicaid program represents such a large share of their revenues.

It is also likely that some of the proposals would require higher outlays by the Medicaid program in certain states. Despite the Boren Amendment, there are states that have managed to keep payment levels relatively low. The effects of any proposal on quality and access to care would be more difficult to assess since they may depend heavily on characteristics of local hospital and nursing home markets.

CONCLUSION

It is hardly surprising that statutory language as vague as "reasonable and adequate to meet the costs which must be incurred by efficiently and economically operated facilities" has produced a spate of litigation. The surprise is that this litigation engine took ten years to build up a good head of steam. Now that the consequences are obvious, it is time to consider whether reform, potentially a variant of one of the options described, should be enacted.

The fundamental questions are what constitutes an adequate payment rate and who should determine if that rate is being paid. It is not clear whether the same policies should apply to nursing homes and hospitals. Similar sets of issues would apply to Medicaid payment rates for physicians' services, hospital outpatient services, drugs, and other services that are not covered by the Medicaid program. More analysis is necessary to develop a set of principles to guide Medicaid payment policy.

REFERENCES AND NOTES

1. There has never been an explicit standard for Medicaid rates for physicians. A number of states have kept these rates low and often have not adjusted them for long periods of time. The refusal of many physicians to treat Medicaid patients has been well documented.

2. Detailed summaries of the major cases are presented in American Public Welfare Association, "Exerpts from the MMI Bulletin Regarding Medicaid Boren Amendment Court Cases Since 1987," *MMI Bulletin* (Washington, D.C.: December 1991); Anderson, G.F., and M.A. Hall, "The Adequacy of Hospital Reimbursement Under Public Medicaid's Boren Amendment," *Journal of Legal Medicine*, 1992, 13:205–236; and Harris, J., *The Boren Amendment: Medicaid Reimbursement to Hospitals and Nursing Facilities, An Issue Brief* (Washington, D.C.: American Public Welfare Association, 1990).

3. Prospective Payment Assessment Commission, *Medicaid Hospital Payment: Congressional Report* (Washington, D.C: C–91–02, October 1, 1991).

PART 3

•
•
•

Federal and State Roles in Financing

5

●

State Medicaid Expansion
in the Early 1990s:
Program Growth in a Period
of Fiscal Stress

VICTOR J. MILLER

INTRODUCTION

The American system of federalism continually undergoes a process of rebalancing and accommodation, and relationships among all levels of government vary with exigency and time. Cities, counties, and other local governments provide most services and are creatures of and subject to the constitutions of their states. State governments are at least nominally sovereign under our constitution. They have independent police powers, including the power to tax, and it is the extent of their delegation of those powers to local governments that determines much of the intergovernmental battleground in most states.

The federal government, originally the creature of the states, is increasingly the preeminent power, even in some areas traditionally reserved for local decision-making. The federal government sometimes deals with state and local governments as equal partners in the governmental enterprise, sometimes as junior partners, and sometimes as administrative entities for delivering federally driven services. And it is the act of transferring funds to state and local governments in the form of "grants-in-aid" that creates the major opportunity for an expansion of the federal presence.

In 1991, 11.5 percent of federal spending consisted of grants-in-aid to state and local governments, the lowest share since the 1960s. These grants varied widely in function, scope, structure, and purpose. They were also perceived very differently by the different levels of government involved.

From the federal perspective, grants-in-aid constitute spending "by the Federal Government in support of state and local programs of government operations or provision of service to the public (1)." Grant programs include entitlements [primarily Medicaid, child nutrition, and Aid to Families with Dependent Children (AFDC)], block grants, shared revenues, in-kind grants, grants to Indian tribes, categorical formula grants, and discretionary grants. Excluded is federal procurement of research services at state universities. Some grants support state programs, some local programs, some local programs under a state plan, and some private programs under a state or local government plan.

From the state perspective, however, these are often understood to be federal programs that use state or local governments as delivery mechanisms and with which states have little choice but to comply. The differing perspectives produce very different conclusions as to (1) program objectives and (2) which governments' objectives are driving the others'.

In reality, grant programs generally support programs of shared interest between the federal government and other governments. In that sense, the federal government does not provide grants because it likes state and local governments, but rather because it wants these governments to share its interests and concerns and to work toward similar ends. And, in particular, it focuses on those governments that would not or could not perform the kind or degree of such work without federal involvement.

As circumstances change, the extent of shared interest changes, and program structures that may have seemed appropriate in one context grow questionable in another. The extraordinary growth of Medicaid in the late 1980s and early 1990s, combined with funding limitations placed on most other federal grants, has caused Medicaid to dominate the intergovernmental grant system. Additionally, Medicaid has achieved this dominance outside traditional decision processes, as costs have accelerated substantially beyond levels projected in either federal or state budget debates, and as the entitlement nature of the program has automatically generated appropriations.

It is the indefinite exposure to Medicaid costs that has legislative appropriations and tax committees uneasy at both federal and state levels. A legislature can limit AFDC costs through restricting eligibility or cutting benefits. It has many fewer options vis-a-vis Medicaid. It is *mandated* to cover many persons with low incomes; it *must* provide reimbursable reimbursement to providers; and so forth.

This Medicaid dominance is projected to continue and increase into the foreseeable future, absent a major program restructuring. As its growth continues, the locus of decision-making will continue to shift away from the traditional political actors to medical and insurance experts both in government and in the insurance and provider communities. It is far from clear that decisions made in this context will be in the best interest of those Medicaid was designed to serve—the poor.

GRANTS-IN-AID: A HISTORICAL PERSPECTIVE (2)

Today's structure of grants-in-aid is generally traced back to the first Morrill Act of 1862. That Act authorized grants of federal lands to the states, which could then raise resources for institutions of higher education by selling these tracts. The Act established three conditions that still govern federal grants-in-aid:

- *National Purpose.* The land grant colleges were to educate the young in "agricultural and mechanical arts," and, given Civil War–related needs, to provide military instruction.

- *Financial Accountability.* States were to invest proceeds of the sales in approved securities.

- *Output.* The states specifically were to provide for instruction.

However, many provisions that might accompany a present-day grant-in-aid program were missing—matching requirements, program plans, cost allocation plans, audits, among others.

In 1887, the Hatch Act provided for the first *annual* grants to states for agricultural experiment stations. States were required to submit annual reports to the U.S. Secretary of the Treasury, and soon thereafter Congress authorized the Secretary of Agriculture to conduct audits. The Smith-Lever Act (1914) established the first *formula* grant in support of state agricultural extension programs, and the Smith-Hughes Act (1917), supporting vocational education, required detailed *planning and administrative requirements.* The first truly large-scale assistance program was enacted in 1916 in the form of federal aid for state highway construction. This was followed by the Vocational Rehabilitation Act of 1920, which helped disabled veterans, and the Sheppard-Towner (Maternity) Act of 1921, which was aimed at decreasing maternal and infant mortality. By the early 1920s, federal grants for highway construction exceeded $90 million each year, with other grants totaling about $26 million.

Emergency Relief

The amount of federal grant-in-aid activity was broadened and deepened with the Great Depression. Billions of dollars in "emergency relief" supported highway, road, and bridge construction, emergency work relief, and emergency expenditures for public bodies. In the peak year of 1935, an astounding total of $2.2 billion (one third of the federal budget) was spent through these programs. Though these programs all terminated as World War II began, they did establish two precedents: (1) the allocation of funds among states on the basis of fiscal capacity and financial burden, and (2) the use of federal grants as part of a program to stimulate the economy.

A further impact of the Depression was the expansion of direct contacts between the federal government and local governments. The Depression left many cities with large unemployed populations and tax delinquencies, and cities banded together successfully to lobby the federal government for direct aid. It was during this period that the federal-local program for public housing was established.

Perhaps the most lasting impact of the Depression on the grant-in-aid system was created by the passage of the Social Security Act of 1935. The Act established many programs whose legislative descendants still provide assistance—programs for old age assistance, aid to the blind, aid to dependent children, unemployment compensation, maternal and child health, crippled children, and child welfare. These programs were large in scope and had substantially larger planning requirements and federal oversight. By World War II, grants for social welfare exceeded construction grants.

Post War World II (1954)

After World War II, new urban-oriented programs continued to be established, including airport construction (1946), urban renewal (1949), and urban planning (1954). However, the most significant grant-in-aid event of the 1950s was the passage of the Highway Act of 1956, which established the Interstate Highway System.

Most new programs of this decade were oriented toward capital investment, and by the 1960s grants for construction once again exceeded those for individuals.

The grant system continued to grow in the 1960s, as governments at all levels supported an expanded governmental presence and as conclusions were reached that the federal government's tax and administrative systems were more appropriate for many programs.

Probably the most important grant-in-aid event of the decade was the addition of Title XIX (Medicaid) to the Social Security Act. A second major event of the 1960s was the passage of the Elementary and Secondary Education Act, which for the first time provided substantial federal resources to help local school districts educate the poor. Overall, the Johnson Administration presided over what the Advisory Commission on Intergovernmental Relations (ACIR) termed an "explosion" in categorical grants. The 1967 ACIR study, *Fiscal Balance in the American Federal System* (3), described the following changes:

- A proliferation of grants,

- An expanded use of project grants,

- An increased variety of matching ratios,

- The development of incentive grants,

- The development of multifunctional grants,

- A diversification of eligible grant recipients,

- Increasing grants to urban areas,

- Inflexibility of administrative and fiscal requirements,

- An expansion of planning requirements, and

- Variation in regional office structures.

The ACIR counted 160 grant authorizations in 1962, and 379 in 1966, most of which were discretionary project grants. Federal grants began bypassing both state and local governments to newly created community action agencies, as the federal government began creating its own quasi-governments. In addition, multifaceted grants with multiple objectives became more prevalent as the federal government attempted programmatically broad attempts to help depressed areas (e.g., model cities, Appalachian regional development) or given clienteles (e.g., Juvenile Delinquency and Youth Offenses Control Act, Older Americans Act, the Economic Opportunity Act). This expansion and diversification of programs was accompanied by an extraordinary increase in state and area-wide planning requirements, and many new federal grants were specifically aimed at underwriting the costs of state bureaucracies to write those plans.

A substantial change in emphasis occurred during this period. While previous grant proposals had resulted from interest at the state and local levels, by the 1960s the federal government itself became the driving force behind establishing and expanding the system. This activism was founded on two premises: (1) that a number of states either could not or would not provide needed services to the poor and to cities, and (2) that the extraordinary revenue-producing capacity of the federal income tax was producing a "fiscal drag" on the economy.

A reaction to this proliferation set in by the 1970s. The Nixon Administration, complaining about "overlapping and duplicative" categorical grants, proposed six "special revenue sharing" programs to replace a myriad of categorical programs. Three of these proposals received some support in Congress, resulting in the enactment of community development block grants (CDBG) and the Comprehensive Employment and Training Act (CETA), and amendments to Law Enforcement Assistance Administration (LEAA) programs. The Administration also proposed substantial AFDC and Medicaid amendments, though the reforms proposed were not seriously entertained by the Congress. In addition, the Administration gave its support to the idea of revenue sharing to assist state and local governments while reducing fiscal drag, and the program was enacted in 1972. The massive growth in grants for education, employment and training, and fiscal assistance shifted the focus of grant spending, with grants for individuals growing more slowly and grants for capital investment shrinking in importance.

Table 1 illustrates the increase in grants through the early 1970s and the maintenance of high levels through most of the decade (4).

The Nixon Administration did not initially step back from its financial commitment to state and local governments. However, faced with deficits exceeding $20 billion and the ongoing enactment of additional budget authority by Congress, the Administration began to administratively im-

Table 1. Grants-in-Aid to state and local governments in the federal budget (federal fiscal years; outlays in millions).

Year	Grants	Budget	Share	% Change in Share
1970	$24.1	$195.6	12.3%	12.0%
1971	28.1	210.2	13.4%	8.7%
1972	$34.4	$230.7	14.9%	11.5%
1973	41.8	245.7	17.0%	14.3%
1974	43.4	269.4	16.1%	-5.5%
1975	49.8	332.3	15.0%	-6.9%
1976	59.1	371.8	15.9%	6.1%
TQ	15.9	96.0	16.6%	4.4%
1977	68.4	409.2	16.7%	0.8%
1978	77.9	458.7	17.0%	1.6%
1979	82.9	503.5	16.5%	-3.1%
1980	91.5	590.9	15.5%	-6.0%
1981	94.8	678.2	14.0%	-9.7%
1982	88.2	745.8	11.8%	-15.4%
1983	92.5	808.4	11.4%	-3.2%
1984	97.6	851.8	11.5%	0.1%
1985	105.9	946.4	11.2%	-2.3%
1986	112.4	990.3	11.3%	1.4%
1987	108.4	1,003.9	10.8%	-4.8%
1988	115.4	1,064.1	10.8%	0.4%
1989	122.0	1,144.2	10.7%	-1.7%
1990	135.4	1,251.8	10.8%	1.4%
1991	152.0	1,323.0	11.5%	6.2%
1992	182.2	1,475.4	12.3%	7.5%
1993	199.1	1,515.3	13.1%	6.4%
1994	200.1	1,475.4	13.6%	3.2%
1995	235.5	1,536.0	15.3%	13.1%
1996	255.1	1,608.1	15.9%	3.5%
1997	275.2	1,684.3	16.3%	3.0%

Source: Budget of the United States Government, February 1992.

pound substantial funds, primarily grants for wastewater treatment and for highway construction. It justified these impoundments on the basis of fiscal policy. Congress, frustrated over its lack of control, passed the Congressional Budget and Impoundment Control Act of 1974. This Act gave Congress the mechanism to establish its own fiscal policy, gave it an independent source of budget data and analysis (the Congressional Budget Office), and required the Executive Branch to ask for permission to not spend appropriated funds.

Congress rejected the Nixon Administration's proposals to defer spending for the grant programs (5), and the commitment to increased spending for grants continued through the Ford and into the Carter Administrations.

As a result, spending for grants continued to double every five years: $15 billion in 1967, $34 billion in 1972, $68 billion in 1977. As a share of total federal spending, grants grew from under 10 percent in 1967 to 15 percent in 1972 to 17 percent in 1977 and 1978 (6).

In the second half of the 1970s, the focus of federal aid shifted toward the Depression-era concept of stimulating the economy through grants to local governments. First in the Ford Administration, and then at the beginning of the Carter Administration, billions of dollars were appropriated for CETA public sector employment, local public works construction of the Economic Development Administration (EDA), and antirecession fiscal assistance (ARFA). From 1976 through 1979, almost $22 billion was appropriated for these programs, almost all of which went directly to local governments, by passing states. This spending was aimed both at economic stimulus and assisting local governments in providing services.

THE DECADE OF RETRENCHMENT

By 1979, the Carter Administration saw potential deficits approaching $100 billion and was faced with a newly skeptical Congress doubtful about the return from this outpouring of grants. As a result, no additional funds were appropriated for ARFA or the EDA local public works program, grants for wastewater treatment and public service employment were cut back, and funding for the state share of general revenue sharing was terminated. This dramatic increase and decline in grant funding proved a watershed, and the subsequent Reagan Administration acted to continue these already substantial reductions. Table 1 illustrates the annual decline in the importance of grants, beginning in 1979.

The Reagan Administration saw four major focuses in grants-in-aid—a continued retreat from direct relationships with local governments, a merging of categorical grants into block grants, increased funds for transportation grants, and reductions in funding for other programs. In addition, new budget law laid the groundwork for the dominance of Medicaid and other programs of aid for individuals.

The passage of the Omnibus Budget Reconciliation Act of 1981 (OBRA 1981) dramatically restructured the grant-in-aid universe. New health, education, and community services block grants to the states replaced categorical grants to state and local governments at severely reduced authorizations. Eligibility for income support programs was restricted, and many existing discretionary programs saw their authorizations for appropriation reduced.

Section 2161 of OBRA 1981 reduced reimbursements to states for Medicaid for three years. Total grants for each state were to be reduced 3.0, 4.0, and 4.5 percent for 1982, 1983, and 1984, respectively. If fully implemented, these reductions would have reduced the federal government's Medicaid share to New York, for example, from 50 percent to 48.5 percent,

48 percent, and 47.75 percent. A state could avoid one percentage point of these losses in three different ways: by having an effective rate setting commission, by having an unemployment rate at least 50 percent higher than the national average, or by achieving sufficient reductions in fraud and abuse. In addition, states whose Medicaid growth was slower than national target levels received "incentive payments" back the following year. Some states acted to avoid losses, and lost little. Others lost the full amount.

OBRA 1981 also contained a provision requiring states to provide extra Medicaid reimbursement to hospitals "which serve a disproportionate number of low income patients with special needs." No definition of "disproportionate" was provided. This provision, though not implemented immediately by the U.S. Department of Health and Human Services (HHS), would later provide a future vehicle through which states could funnel substantial amounts of reimbursements to a variety of hospitals and other providers.

Subsequent to OBRA 1981, the passage of the Job Training Partnership Act (JTPA) eliminated public service employment as a federally subsidized activity. Later, general revenue sharing was terminated at least partially because it made payments to all jurisdictions regardless of need. Appropriations for community development grants were severely cut back, and wastewater treatment grants saw both reductions in funding and a restructuring from local grants into state revolving funds. As a result of these and other shifts, budget authority (7) for grants dropped over 13 percent in 1982.

Almost immediately, though, Congress responded to a severe recession by replacing part of the lost appropriations. Approximately $4 billion in grant funds was allocated through the 1983 emergency "jobs bill" supplemental appropriation. Unlike previous efforts at economic stimulation, these funds were disbursed through a wide variety of existing programs. However, most allocation formulas were amended to include an unemployment component, and the state-by-state distribution of funds, though not perfect, did tend to favor governments in states with higher unemployment rates.

The Reagan Administration initially placed a major emphasis on increasing transportation grants. An increase in the gasoline tax from 4 to 9 cents per gallon significantly increased funds flowing into the Highway Trust Fund, beginning in 1983. Budget authority for transportation grants increased from $12.8 billion in 1982 to $18.5 billion in 1983 and $20.2 billion in 1985. Outlays, which lag construction budget authority by 2 to 3 years, also grew in the middle 1980s. However, increasingly severe obligation limitations withheld much of this authority from disbursement, building up balances in the Highway Trust Fund and slowing the increases in program outlays that might otherwise have been expected.

GRAMM-RUDMAN-HOLLINGS AND NEW BUDGETING

The passage of Gramm-Rudman-Hollings (GRH) deficit reduction legislation in 1985 initiated a new era in federal budgeting. GRH set specific deficit targets and mandated across-the-board cuts in budgetary resources (sequesters) to meet those targets. The legislation had three significant impacts on the flow of federal grants. First, it reduced 1986 budget authority for grants by an estimated $3 billion. Second, it produced greater uncertainties, as the bill was passed and implemented by the various grant-making agencies, then declared unconstitutional, then reaffirmed in a restructured format by Congress.

Most important, GRH expressed congressional priorities in its exemptions and special rules. Social Security, other retirement programs, and a group of needs-based entitlements such as Medicaid, AFDC, and child nutrition programs were totally exempted from GRH sequesters, even if their increases caused the cutbacks. Programs such as foster care and Medicare received partial protection. While some programs outside this group received increases, in the latter half of the 1980s most grant-in-aid growth was confined to the GRH safety net.

The GRH mechanism and other budget devices thus became the structure for Medicaid expansions. Budget reconciliation bills, nominally aimed at reconciling entitlement spending down to levels assumed in the budget resolution, became the vehicle for astute legislators to expand their programs. Cuts in one program, such as Medicare, could be used to offset the relatively small first-year costs of major entitlement expansions in a program such as Medicaid.

The enactment in 1990 of the Budget Enforcement Act (BEA) confirmed and reinforced the GRH legacy. Programs previously exempt from sequester remained exempt. However, the BEA effectively eliminated the GRH focus on a deficit target for federal fiscal years 1991–1993 by (1) setting ceilings on discretionary program appropriations, (2) exempting the massive expenditures for the savings and loan industry, and (3) totally ignoring the costs of entitlement programs under current law. Thus, growth in Medicaid could proceed unchecked so long as federal legislation or regulation did not add to it. As a result, grants to state and local governments have begun to grow again as a share of the federal budget, and that growth is projected to continue (see Table 1).

RECENT HISTORY OF GRANTS

Grants by Budget Function

The history described above has produced an ongoing shift in grants for different purposes. Tables 2 and 2a provide one perspective in the changes—grants by federal budget function.

In 1977, the peak year of grants relative to the budget, grants for education, training, employment, and social services (ETESS) programs totaled $15.7 billion (23 percent). Grants were also concentrated in the

Table 2. Functional history of federal Grants-in-Aid, 1977–1997 (federal fiscal years; outlays in millions).

	1977	1979	1981	1983	1985	1987	1989	1991	1993 est.	1997 proj.	Percent Change 1977-87	1987-91	1991-93	1993-97
National Defense	$96	$94	$75	$86	$157	$193	$253	$185	$114	$131	101.0%	-4.1%	-38.4%	14.9%
Energy	74	183	617	482	529	455	420	457	439	446	514.9%	0.4%	-3.9%	1.6%
Natural Resources & Environment	4,189	4,631	4,944	4,018	4,069	4,073	3,606	4,040	3,962	3,184	-2.8%	-0.8%	-1.9%	-19.6%
Agriculture	371	456	829	1,822	2,420	2,092	1,359	1,220	1,251	1,236	463.9%	-41.7%	2.5%	-1.2%
Commerce & Housing Credit	8	12	4	62	2	1	0	0	0	0	-87.5%	N/A	N/A	N/A
Transportation	8,299	10,438	13,462	13,248	17055	16,919	18,225	19,878	22,333	22,529	103.9%	17.5%	12.4%	0.9%
Community & Regional Development	4,496	6,641	6,124	4,962	5,221	4,235	4,074	4,273	4,915	3,696	-5.8%	0.9%	15.0%	-24.8%
Education, Trng, Employ & Soc Svcs	15,753	22,249	21,474	16,125	17,817	18,657	21,987	26,020	29,851	32,619	18.4%	39.5%	14.7%	9.3%
Health	12,104	14,377	18,895	20,224	24,451	29,466	36,679	55,783	88,500	155,074	143.4%	89.3%	58.7%	75.2%
Income Security	12,663	14,740	21,013	24,758	27,153	29,972	32,523	36,856	44,133	52,674	136.7%	23.0%	19.7%	19.4%
Veterans Benefits & Services	79	86	74	66	91	95	127	141	217	194	20.3%	48.4%	53.9%	-10.6%
Administration of Justice	713	517	332	101	95	288	520	940	1,118	1,068	-59.6%	226.4%	18.9%	-4.5%
General Government	9,571	8,434	6,918	6,541	6,838	2,000	2,204	2,224	2,282	2,317	-79.1%	11.2%	2.6%	1.5%
Total	$68,415	$82,858	$94,762	$92,495	$105,897	$108,446	$121,976	$152,017	$199,116	$275,167	58.5%	40.2%	31.0%	38.2%
Memorandum:														
Health	12,104	14,377	18,895	20,224	24,451	29,466	36,679	55,783	88,500	155,074	143.4%	89.3%	58.7%	75.2%
All Other	56,311	68,481	75,867	72,271	81,446	78,980	85,297	96,234	110,616	120,093	40.3%	21.8%	14.9%	8.6%

Source: Budget of the United States Government, February 1992.

Table 2a. Percent functional history of federal Grants-in-Aid, 1977–1991 (federal fiscal years).

	1977	1979	1981	1983	1985	1987	1989	1991	1993 est.	1997 proj.	Percent Change			
											1977-87	1987-91	1991-93	1991-93
National Defense	0.1%	0.1%	0.1%	0.1%	0.1%	0.2%	0.2%	0.1%	0.1%	0.0%	26.8%	-31.6%	-53.0%	-16.8%
Energy	0.1%	0.2%	0.7%	0.5%	0.5%	0.4%	0.3%	0.3%	0.2%	0.2%	287.9%	-28.3%	-26.7%	-26.5%
Natural Resources & Environment	6.1%	5.6%	5.2%	4.3%	3.8%	3.8%	3.0%	2.7%	2.0%	1.2%	-38.7%	-29.2%	-25.1%	-41.8%
Agriculture	0.5%	0.6%	0.9%	2.0%	2.3%	1.9%	1.1%	0.8%	0.6%	0.4%	255.7%	-58.4%	-21.7%	-28.5%
Commerce & Housing Credit	0.0%	0.0%	0.0%	0.1%	0.0%	0.0%	0.0%	0.0%	0.0%	0.0%	-92.1%	N/A	N/A	N/A
Transportation	12.1%	12.6%	14.2%	14.3%	16.1%	15.6%	14.9%	13.1%	11.2%	8.2%	28.6%	-16.2%	-14.2%	-27.0%
Community & Regional Development	6.6%	8.0%	6.5%	5.4%	4.9%	3.9%	3.3%	2.8%	2.5%	1.3%	-40.6%	-28.0%	-12.2%	-45.6%
Education, Trng, Employ & Soc Svcs	23.0%	26.9%	22.7%	17.4%	16.8%	17.2%	18.0%	17.1%	15.0%	11.9%	-25.3%	-0.5%	-12.4%	-20.9%
Health	17.7%	17.4%	19.9%	21.9%	23.1%	27.2%	30.1%	36.7%	44.4%	56.4%	53.6%	35.1%	21.1%	26.8%
Income Security	18.5%	17.8%	22.2%	26.8%	25.6%	27.6%	26.7%	24.2%	22.2%	19.1%	49.3%	-12.3%	-8.6%	-13.6%
Veterans Benefits & Services	0.1%	0.1%	0.1%	0.1%	0.1%	0.1%	0.1%	0.1%	0.1%	0.1%	-24.1%	5.9%	17.5%	-35.3%
Administration of Justice	1.0%	0.6%	0.4%	0.1%	0.1%	0.3%	0.4%	0.6%	0.6%	0.4%	-74.5%	132.8%	-9.2%	-30.9%
General Government	14.0%	10.2%	7.3%	7.1%	6.5%	1.8%	1.8%	1.5%	1.1%	0.8%	-86.8%	-20.7%	-21.7%	-26.5%
Total	100.0%	100.0%	100.0%	100.0%	100.0%	100.0%	100.0%	100.0%	100.0%	100.0%	0.0%	0.0%	0.0%	0.0%
Memorandum:														
Health	17.7%	17.4%	19.9%	21.9%	23.1%	27.2%	30.1%	36.7%	44.4%	56.4%	53.6%	35.1%	21.1%	26.8%
All Other	82.3%	82.6%	80.1%	78.1%	76.9%	72.8%	69.9%	63.3%	55.6%	43.6%	-11.5%	-13.1%	-12.2%	-21.4%

following functions: income security, $12.7 billion (18.5 percent); health, $12.1 billion (17.7 percent); general government, $9.6 billion (14.0 percent); and transportation, $8.3 billion (12.1 percent).

In the following ten years, the elimination of general revenue sharing and most LEAA spending substantially reduced general government and justice grants, and the elimination of CETA offset education growth in the ETESS function. Both health and income security grants more than doubled. By 1987, health and income security grants were 55 percent of the total.

Since 1987, however, growth in health grants has accelerated. Health grants grew 17 percent per year in the period 1987–1991 and are estimated to grow more than 25 percent per year in 1991–1993. By comparison, the projected 15 percent per year increase to 1997 seems tame. By 1989 health grants had increased to 30.1 percent of the total, with further increases to 36.7 percent in 1991 and a projected 44.4 percent in 1993. Only the relatively small programs for veterans (primarily for medical care) and for law enforcement (anti-drug abuse) will have kept pace.

By 1997, the budget projects that health grants will grow to 56.4 percent of grants. If these projections prove true, grants would total $275 billion in 1997. This would constitute 16.3 percent of the budget, a share not equaled since the growth days of the late 1970s.

Grants by Type

The growth in grants is dominated by what are termed "payments for individuals," transfer programs that provide financial assistance to state and local governments to aid specific categories of individuals (8). Tables 3 and 3a illustrate the growth in Medicaid and other such programs through 1985. Payments for individuals, primarily AFDC, constituted about half of federal grants after World War II and remained dominant until the second half of the 1960s. This dominance was reduced by the creation of the federal-aid highways program. However, the growth of both Medicaid and child nutrition programs in the 1980–1985 period reversed the decline. By 1985, payments for individuals constituted as dominant a share of the grant system as in 1945.

Tables 4 and 4a bring this experience up to date. By 1993, payments for individuals are estimated to be 64.5 percent of grants, with Medicaid two thirds of that amount. By 1997, Medicaid alone is projected to be 54.8 percent of grants, and total payments for individuals are projected to be 74.2 percent of the total.

By comparison, grants for capital expenditures are projected to fall from 15 percent of grants in 1993 to 11 percent in 1997. Despite the much-heralded new highway program, grants for transportation would fall from 11 to 8 percent. Despite the much-bewailed problems of the cities, grants for community and regional development would fall from 2 to 1 percent of the total. Even ever popular education grants would fall as a share of the total, victim of inexorable budget controls for discretionary appropriations.

Table 3. Historical grants to state and local government for different purposes (federal fiscal years; dollars in millions).

| | 1945 | 1950 | 1955 | 1960 | 1965 | 1970 | 1975 | 1980 | 1985 | Percent Change | | | |
										1945-60	1960-70	1970-80	1980-85
Payments for Individuals:													
Medicaid	$0	$0	$0	$0	$272	$2,727	$6,840	$13,957	$22,655	N/A	N/A	411.8%	62.3%
Nutrition Programs	0	83	84	232	295	938	2,152	5,074	7,431	N/A	N/A	440.9%	46.4%
AFDC and Related Programs	401	1,123	1,438	2,059	2,787	4,142	5,231	8,107	10,731	412.9%	101.2%	95.7%	32.4%
Foster Care/Adoption Assistance	0	0	0	0	0	0	0	0	738	N/A	N/A	N/A	N/A
Subsidized Housing	9	7	67	127	208	442	1,333	3,453	6,417	1364.4%	246.9%	681.2%	85.8%
Other	1	3	5	6	8	17	48	465	580	500.0%	183.3%	2635.3%	24.7%
Subtotal, Payments for Indiv	411	1,217	1,593	2,424	3,570	8,266	15,605	31,056	48,552	489.7%	241.0%	275.7%	56.3%
Capital Investment:													
Transportation	33	465	594	2,984	4,079	4,514	5,568	11,580	15,921	8942.4%	51.3%	156.5%	37.5%
Community & Regional Develop	119	1	40	106	582	1,624	2,494	5,787	4,997	-10.9%	1432.1%	256.3%	-13.7%
Natural Resources & Environm	1	6	21	88	159	365	2,276	4,906	3,602	8700.0%	314.8%	1244.1%	-26.6%
Other	0	12	165	143	165	553	543	211	355	N/A	286.7%	-61.8%	68.2%
Subtotal, Capital Investment	153	484	820	3,321	4,985	7,056	10,881	22,484	24,875	2070.6%	112.5%	218.7%	10.6%
Other Programs:													
Education 1/	69	39	243	358	599	2,943	4,193	6,617	7,151	418.8%	722.1%	124.8%	8.1%
General Government	6	37	105	165	226	479	7,072	8,616	6,838	2655.0%	189.6%	1699.9%	-20.6%
Employment and Training 2/	96	208	194	317	486	1,578	3,975	9,904	5,295	230.0%	397.6%	527.6%	-46.5%
Other	123	270	253	434	1,044	3,743	8,066	12,774	13,186	251.5%	762.9%	241.3%	3.2%
Subtotal, Other Programs	295	553	795	1,274	2,355	8,743	23,306	37,911	32,470	332.7%	586.1%	333.6%	-14.4%
Total	$859	$2,253	$3,207	$7,019	$10,910	$24,065	$49,791	$91,451	$105,897	717.5%	242.8%	280.0%	15.8%
Memorandum:													
Grants as share of Budget	0.9%	5.3%	4.7%	7.6%	9.2%	12.3%	15.0%	15.5%	11.2%	722.2%	61.5%	25.6%	-27.7%

1/ Includes all programs now administered by the U.S. Department of Education except rehabilitation services and student aid.
2/ Includes grants for administration of the unemployment insurance system.

Table 3a. Percentage historical grants to state and local government for different purposes (federal fiscal years).

	1945	1950	1955	1960	1965	1970	1975	1980	1985	Percent Change 1945-60	1960-70	1970-80	1980-85
Payments for Individuals:													
Medicaid	0.0%	0.0%	0.0%	0.0%	2.5%	11.3%	13.7%	15.3%	21.4%	N/A	N/A	34.7%	40.2%
Nutrition Programs	0.0%	3.7%	2.6%	3.3%	2.7%	3.9%	4.3%	5.5%	7.0%	N/A	N/A	42.3%	26.5%
AFDC and Related Programs	46.8%	49.9%	44.8%	29.3%	25.5%	17.2%	10.5%	8.9%	10.1%	-37.3%	-41.3%	-48.5%	14.3%
Foster Care/Adoption Assistance	0.0%	0.0%	0.0%	0.0%	0.0%	0.0%	0.0%	0.0%	0.7%	N/A	N/A	N/A	N/A
Subsidized Housing	1.0%	0.3%	2.1%	1.8%	1.9%	1.8%	2.7%	3.8%	6.1%	79.1%	1.2%	105.6%	60.5%
Other	0.1%	0.1%	0.2%	0.1%	0.1%	0.1%	0.1%	0.5%	0.5%	-26.6%	-17.4%	619.8%	7.7%
Subtotal Payments for Indiv	47.9%	54.0%	49.7%	34.5%	32.7%	34.3%	31.3%	34.0%	45.8%	-27.9%	-0.5%	-1.1%	35.0%
Capital Investment:													
Transportation	3.8%	20.6%	18.5%	42.5%	37.4%	18.8%	11.2%	12.7%	15.0%	1006.1%	-55.9%	-32.5%	18.7%
Community & Regional Develop	13.9%	0.0%	1.2%	1.5%	5.3%	6.7%	5.0%	6.3%	4.7%	-89.1%	346.9%	-6.2%	-25.4%
Natural Resources & Environm	0.1%	0.3%	0.7%	1.3%	1.5%	1.5%	4.6%	5.4%	3.4%	976.4%	21.0%	253.7%	-36.6%
Other	0.0%	0.5%	5.1%	2.0%	1.5%	2.3%	1.1%	0.2%	0.3%	N/A	12.8%	-90.0%	45.3%
Subtotal Capital Investment	17.8%	21.5%	25.6%	47.3%	45.7%	29.3%	21.9%	24.6%	23.5%	165.5%	-38.0%	-16.1%	-4.5%
Other Programs:													
Elem, Sec, and Vocat Education	8.0%	1.7%	7.6%	5.1%	5.5%	12.2%	8.4%	7.2%	6.8%	-36.5%	139.8%	-40.8%	-6.7%
General Government	0.7%	1.6%	3.3%	2.4%	2.1%	2.0%	14.2%	9.4%	6.5%	237.0%	-15.5%	373.6%	-31.5%
Employment and Training	11.2%	9.2%	6.0%	4.5%	4.5%	6.6%	8.0%	10.8%	5.0%	-59.6%	45.2%	65.2%	-53.8%
Other	14.4%	12.0%	7.9%	6.2%	9.6%	15.6%	16.2%	14.0%	12.5%	-57.0%	151.7%	-10.2%	-10.9%
Subtotal Other Programs	34.3%	24.5%	24.8%	18.2%	21.6%	36.3%	46.8%	41.5%	30.7%	-47.1%	100.1%	14.1%	-26.0%
Total	100.0%	100.0%	100.0%	100.0%	100.0%	100.0%	100.0%	100.0%	100.0%	0.0%	0.0%	0.0%	0.0%

Table 4. Recent history of grants to state and local government for different purposes (federal fiscal years; dollars in millions).

	1985	1986	1987	1988	1989	1990	1991	1992 est.	1993 budget	1997 budget	Annual Percent Change			
											1985-90	990-92	1992-93	993-97
Payments for Individuals:														
Medicaid	$22,655	$24,996	$27,435	$30,462	$34,604	$41,103	$52,533	$72,503	$84,396	$150,665	16.1%	32.8%	16.4%	15.6%
Nutrition Programs	7,431	7,707	8,267	8,688	9,323	9,939	10,953	12,169	12,660	15,201	7.5%	10.7%	4.0%	4.7%
AFDC and Related Programs	10,731	11,922	12,369	12,349	12,559	13,560	15,262	16,831	16,764	18,544	6.0%	11.4%	-0.4%	2.6%
Foster Care/Adoption Assistance	738	794	783	988	1,338	1,579	2,120	2,500	2,835	4,608	20.9%	25.8%	13.4%	12.9%
Subsidized Housing	6,417	7,443	7,400	8,651	8,553	9,552	7,913	9,342	10,978	14,802	10.5%	-1.1%	17.5%	7.8%
Other	580	585	534	495	884	1,139	1,251	1,037	855	421	18.4%	-4.6%	-17.6%	-16.2%
Subtotal, Payments for Indiv	48,552	53,447	56,788	61,633	67,261	76,872	90,032	114,382	126,688	204,241	12.2%	22.0%	12.3%	12.3%
Capital Investment:														
Transportation	15,921	17,539	15,966	16,956	17,057	18,338	18,964	20,411	21,531	21,720	3.6%	5.5%	5.5%	0.2%
Community & Regional Develop	4,997	4,531	3,998	4,046	3,894	3,739	3,736	3,988	4,114	3,094	-7.0%	3.3%	3.2%	-6.9%
Natural Resources & Environm	3,602	3,812	3,567	3,257	3,098	3,267	3,475	3,339	3,295	2,648	-2.4%	1.1%	-1.3%	-5.3%
Other	355	378	312	359	492	461	355	404	659	1,709	6.8%	-6.4%	63.1%	26.9%
Subtotal, Capital Investment	24,875	26,260	23,843	24,618	24,541	25,805	26,530	28,142	29,599	29,171	0.9%	4.4%	5.2%	-0.4%
Other Programs:														
Education 1/	7,151	7,514	7,347	7,977	8,698	9,471	10,603	12,339	13,116	14,328	7.3%	14.1%	6.3%	2.2%
General Government	6,838	7,158	2,000	1,950	2,204	2,309	2,224	2,313	2,282	2,317	-23.8%	0.1%	-1.3%	0.4%
Employment and Training 2/	5,295	5,616	5,496	5,608	5,792	5,894	6,089	6,881	6,747	6,491	2.7%	8.0%	-1.9%	-1.0%
Other	13,186	12,385	12,972	13,596	13,480	15,026	16,539	18,153	18,884	18,619	3.3%	9.9%	4.0%	-0.4%
Subtotal, Other Programs	32,470	32,673	27,815	29,131	30,176	32,700	35,455	39,686	41,029	41,755	0.2%	10.2%	3.4%	0.4%
Total	$105,897	$112,379	$108,446	$115,382	$121,976	$135,377	$152,017	$182,210	$199,116	$275,167	6.3%	16.0%	9.3%	8.4%
Memorandum:														
Grants as Share of Budget	11.2%	11.3%	10.8%	10.8%	10.7%	10.8%	11.5%	12.3%	13.1%	16.3%	-0.8%	6.9%	6.4%	5.6%

1/ Includes all programs now administered by the U.S. Department of Education except rehabilitation services and student aid.
2/ Includes grants for administration of the unemployment insurance system.

Table 4a. Recent percent history of grants to state and local government for different purposes (federal fiscal years).

	1985	1986	1987	1988	1989	1990	1991	1992 est.	1993 budget	1997 budget	Annual Percent Change			
											1985-90	990-92	1992-93	993-97
Payments for Individuals:														
Medicaid	21.4%	22.2%	25.3%	26.4%	28.4%	30.4%	34.6%	39.8%	42.4%	54.8%	9.1%	14.5%	6.5%	6.6%
Nutrition Programs	7.0%	6.9%	7.6%	7.5%	7.6%	7.3%	7.2%	6.7%	6.4%	5.5%	1.1%	-4.6%	-4.8%	-3.5%
AFDC and Related Programs	10.1%	10.6%	11.4%	10.7%	10.3%	10.0%	10.0%	9.2%	8.4%	6.7%	-0.3%	-4.0%	-8.9%	-5.4%
Foster Care/Adoption Assistance	0.7%	0.7%	0.7%	0.9%	1.1%	1.2%	1.4%	1.4%	1.4%	1.7%	13.7%	8.5%	3.8%	4.1%
Subsidized Housing	6.1%	6.6%	6.8%	7.5%	7.0%	7.1%	5.2%	5.1%	5.5%	5.4%	3.9%	-14.8%	7.5%	-0.6%
Other	0.5%	0.5%	0.5%	0.4%	0.7%	0.8%	0.8%	0.6%	0.4%	0.2%	11.3%	-17.8%	-24.6%	-22.7%
Subtotal, Payments for Indiv	45.8%	47.6%	52.4%	53.4%	55.1%	56.8%	59.2%	62.8%	64.5%	74.2%	5.5%	5.1%	2.8%	3.6%
Capital Investment:														
Transportation	15.0%	15.6%	14.7%	14.7%	14.0%	13.5%	12.5%	11.2%	10.8%	7.9%	-2.6%	-9.1%	-3.5%	-7.6%
Community & Regional Develop	4.7%	4.0%	3.7%	3.5%	3.2%	2.8%	2.5%	2.2%	2.1%	1.1%	-12.5%	-11.0%	-5.6%	-14.1%
Natural Resources & Environm	3.4%	3.4%	3.3%	2.8%	2.5%	2.4%	2.3%	1.8%	1.7%	1.0%	-8.2%	-12.9%	-9.7%	-12.7%
Other	0.3%	0.3%	0.3%	0.3%	0.4%	0.3%	0.2%	0.2%	0.3%	0.6%	0.4%	-19.3%	49.3%	17.0%
Subtotal, Capital Investment	23.5%	23.4%	22.0%	21.3%	20.1%	19.1%	17.5%	15.4%	14.9%	10.6%	-5.1%	10.0%	-3.8%	-8.1%
Other Programs:														
Elem, Sec, and Vocat Education	6.8%	6.7%	6.8%	6.9%	7.1%	7.0%	7.0%	6.8%	6.6%	5.2%	0.9%	-1.6%	-2.7%	-5.7%
General Government	6.5%	6.4%	1.8%	1.7%	1.8%	1.7%	1.5%	1.3%	1.1%	0.8%	-28.3%	-13.7%	-9.7%	-7.4%
Employment and Training 1/	5.0%	5.0%	5.1%	4.9%	4.7%	4.4%	4.0%	3.8%	3.4%	2.4%	-3.4%	-6.9%	-10.3%	-8.7%
Other	12.5%	11.0%	12.0%	11.8%	11.1%	11.1%	10.9%	10.0%	9.5%	6.8%	-2.8%	-5.3%	-4.8%	-8.1%
Subtotal, Other Programs	30.7%	29.1%	25.6%	25.2%	24.7%	24.2%	23.3%	21.8%	20.6%	15.2%	-5.8%	-5.0%	-5.4%	-7.4%
Total	100.0%	100.0%	100.0%	100.0%	100.0%	100.0%	100.0%	100.0%	100.0%	100.0%	0.0%	0.0%	0.0%	0.0%

PERSPECTIVES ON STATE AND REGIONAL
DIFFERENCES IN MEDICAID SPENDING

Medicaid as a share of federal grants

The growth in Medicaid grants has been very different among states. Table 5 shows Medicaid outlays by state in 1974, 1980, and the two most recent years for which final data are available, 1990 and 1991. It then compares those outlays to total grant-in-aid outlays.

Medicaid was still a relatively new program in 1974, constituting 12.6 percent of total grants. This share was heavily concentrated in a few, mainly urban states: New York (24 percent), Massachusetts (19 percent), California and Wisconsin (each 17 percent), and Rhode Island, Illinois, Michigan, and Minnesota (15 percent). On a regional basis, the three northeastern regions and the Far West dominated the Medicaid program. For more than half the states, Medicaid produced less than one tenth of their grant-in-aid funds.

By 1980, this situation had changed. Medicaid was over 15 percent of grants. Many of the Southeast, Southwest, Plains, and Rocky Mountain states with small programs four years earlier were experiencing the fastest growth.

By 1991, Medicaid dominated grants for most states, especially in New England (40.2 percent), the Mideast (38.7 percent), and the Southeast (38.5 percent). While New England and Mideast states generally have high societal preferences for governmental services, the dominance in the Southeast has other roots. These include (1) high matching rates (Mississippi receives four federal dollars for state dollar; New York receives one); (2) federal Medicaid mandates requiring southern states to extend Medicaid to their large poverty populations; and (3) a preference in southern states for Medicaid over other forms of public assistance, such as AFDC. Medicaid continues to be a smaller share of total grants for many Western states, which receive large amounts of shared revenues.

MEDICAID AS A SHARE OF STATE AND
LOCAL GOVERNMENT EXPENDITURES

The Census Bureau's *Government Finances* series includes Medicaid spending in a "public welfare" category, making it difficult to isolate Medicaid in state and local government budgets. A separate category, "health and hospitals," reflects spending by state and local governments for the direct provision of services. Tables 6 and 7 compare 1990 (9) government spending by region to a 1977 base.

Public safety spending grew 255 percent over this period, from 7.6 to 8.9 percent of the total. This primarily represents both the construction and operation of prisons. Health and hospital spending also grew substantially from a larger base to 8.9 percent. Public welfare grew marginally, with Medicaid increases presumably offset by reductions in cash assistance.

Table 5. Medicaid as a share of grants to states, 1974–1991 (federal fiscal years; $ in millions).

	1974 Medicaid	1974 Total	1974 Share	1980 Medicaid	1980 Total	1980 Share	Change in Share
New England:	*$423*	*$2,808*	*15.1%*	*$1,051*	*$5,745*	*18.3%*	*21.4%*
CONNECTICUT	68	669	10.2%	192	1,157	16.6%	63.2%
MAINE	36	278	13.0%	107	523	20.5%	57.4%
MASSACHUSETTS	249	1,312	19.0%	559	2,887	19.4%	1.9%
NEW HAMPSHIRE	14	150	9.7%	50	346	14.5%	49.6%
RHODE ISLAND	36	249	14.6%	97	477	20.3%	39.3%
VERMONT	19	151	12.7%	46	356	13.1%	2.7%
Mideast:	*1,802*	*10,407*	*17.3%*	*3,913*	*20,373*	*19.2%*	*10.9%*
DELAWARE	7	119	5.7%	24	275	8.6%	52.1%
DIST OF COL	36	610	5.9%	91	1,336	6.8%	16.3%
MARYLAND	93	750	12.4%	219	1,843	11.9%	-4.2%
NEW JERSEY	159	1,316	12.0%	409	2,833	14.4%	19.9%
NEW YORK	1,241	5,221	23.8%	2,441	9,570	25.5%	7.3%
PENNSYLVANIA	268	2,390	11.2%	730	4,516	16.2%	44.4%
Great Lakes:	*984*	*7,370*	*13.4%*	*2,443*	*15,472*	*15.8%*	*18.3%*
ILLINOIS	330	2,265	14.6%	664	4,477	14.8%	1.9%
INDIANA	76	711	10.7%	237	1,608	14.7%	37.3%
MICHIGAN	264	1,816	14.5%	621	3,929	15.8%	8.7%
OHIO	173	1,760	9.8%	484	3,434	14.1%	43.1%
WISCONSIN	141	818	17.2%	437	2,025	21.6%	25.6%
Plains:	*302*	*3,194*	*9.5%*	*988*	*6,520*	*15.2%*	*60.4%*
IOWA	36	451	8.1%	145	995	14.5%	80.3%
KANSAS	42	385	10.9%	110	818	13.4%	23.3%
MINNESOTA	126	871	14.5%	359	1,667	21.5%	48.4%
MISSOURI	46	853	5.4%	224	1,703	13.1%	143.1%
NEBRASKA	27	272	9.9%	73	547	13.3%	35.0%
NORTH DAKOTA	12	152	8.1%	35	347	10.1%	24.7%
SOUTH DAKOTA	12	210	5.8%	44	443	9.9%	70.3%
Southeast:	*879*	*9,901*	*8.9%*	*2,836*	*19,399*	*14.6%*	*64.6%*
ALABAMA	79	829	9.5%	214	1,584	13.5%	42.2%
ARKANSAS	53	470	11.2%	189	940	20.1%	79.0%
FLORIDA	71	1,161	6.1%	261	2,854	9.2%	49.2%
GEORGIA	135	1,124	12.0%	332	2,373	14.0%	16.0%
KENTUCKY	64	826	7.7%	246	1,471	16.7%	116.8%
LOUISIANA	83	947	8.8%	320	1,568	20.4%	131.7%
MISSISSIPPI	71	686	10.3%	176	1,190	14.8%	43.6%
NORTH CAROLINA	101	975	10.3%	293	1,929	15.2%	47.0%
SOUTH CAROLINA	42	559	7.5%	195	1,068	18.3%	141.8%
TENNESSEE	68	851	8.0%	276	1,696	16.3%	102.2%
VIRGINIA	89	891	10.0%	244	1,775	13.7%	36.9%
WEST VIRGINIA	23	582	3.9%	91	950	9.5%	144.6%
Southwest:	*383*	*3,490*	*11.0%*	*944*	*6,532*	*14.5%*	*31.6%*
ARIZONA	0	427	0.0%	0	838	0.0%	N/A
NEW MEXICO	19	337	5.6%	55	669	8.3%	47.8%
OKLAHOMA	90	598	15.1%	217	1,061	20.4%	35.3%
TEXAS	274	2,128	12.9%	673	3,964	17.0%	31.6%
Rocky Mountain:	*99*	*1,298*	*7.6%*	*261*	*2,741*	*9.5%*	*24.4%*
COLORADO	50	503	10.0%	103	995	10.3%	2.7%
IDAHO	13	187	6.7%	40	393	10.2%	52.0%
MONTANA	12	213	5.7%	43	486	8.8%	54.7%
UTAH	21	275	7.7%	68	572	11.9%	54.6%
WYOMING	3	119	2.5%	7	294	2.5%	2.4%
Far West:	*892*	*6,144*	*14.5%*	*1,871*	*12,051*	*15.5%*	*6.9%*
CALIFORNIA	776	4,666	16.6%	1,526	8,804	17.3%	4.2%
NEVADA	7	127	5.7%	24	335	7.2%	25.1%
OREGON	36	558	6.5%	110	1,237	8.9%	36.0%
WASHINGTON	72	793	9.1%	211	1,674	12.6%	38.0%
ALASKA	4	234	1.8%	22	451	5.0%	183.3%
HAWAII	18	245	7.2%	46	463	9.9%	37.6%
PUERTO RICO	30	543	5.5%	30	1,430	2.1%	-62.0%
TERRITORIES	2	207	0.7%	2	511	0.3%	-54.5%
TOTAL	*$5,818*	*$46,040*	*12.6%*	*$13,957*	*$91,365*	*15.3%*	*20.9%*

Source: U.S. Treasury and Census publications. Totals differ slightly from OMB estimates.

5. (cont). Medicaid as a share of grants to states, 1974–1991 (federal fiscal years; $ in millions)

	1990			1991			Change in Share	
	Medicaid	Total	Share	Medicaid	Total	Share	1990-91	1974-91
New England:	*$2,938*	*$8,169*	*36.0%*	*$3,970*	*$9,884*	*40.2%*	*11.7%*	*166.6%*
CONNECTICUT	613	1,973	31.1%	787	2,393	32.9%	5.8%	223.9%
MAINE	283	762	37.1%	393	926	42.4%	14.2%	226.3%
MASSACHUSETTS	1,570	3,857	40.7%	2,102	4,709	44.6%	9.7%	135.1%
NEW HAMPSHIRE	121	427	28.4%	205	540	38.0%	33.7%	292.1%
RHODE ISLAND	246	773	31.8%	349	908	38.4%	20.7%	163.7%
VERMONT	105	377	27.9%	134	409	32.8%	17.8%	158.2%
Mideast:	*10,281*	*30,244*	*34.0%*	*12,929*	*33,404*	*38.7%*	*13.9%*	*123.5%*
DELAWARE	68	313	21.7%	99	386	25.6%	17.6%	350.5%
DIST OF COL	217	1,718	12.6%	258	1,847	14.0%	10.7%	137.6%
MARYLAND	620	2,350	26.4%	783	2,557	30.6%	16.1%	147.6%
NEW JERSEY	1,261	3,977	31.7%	1,612	4,517	35.7%	12.5%	196.4%
NEW YORK	6,301	15,761	40.0%	7,776	17,226	45.1%	12.9%	90.0%
PENNSYLVANIA	1,814	6,125	29.6%	2,401	6,870	34.9%	18.0%	212.2%
Great Lakes:	*6,577*	*20,380*	*32.3%*	*7,936*	*23,166*	*34.3%*	*6.1%*	*156.6%*
ILLINOIS	1,276	5,280	24.2%	1,431	5,954	24.0%	-0.6%	65.1%
INDIANA	945	2,423	39.0%	1,133	2,767	40.9%	5.0%	282.2%
MICHIGAN	1,506	4,751	31.7%	1,944	5,426	35.8%	13.0%	146.3%
OHIO	1,957	5,388	36.3%	2,356	6,220	37.9%	4.3%	284.7%
WISCONSIN	893	2,538	35.2%	1,072	2,799	38.3%	8.8%	122.9%
Plains:	*2,551*	*8,615*	*29.6%*	*3,474*	*9,966*	*34.9%*	*17.7%*	*268.7%*
IOWA	414	1,289	32.1%	518	1,475	35.1%	9.2%	335.2%
KANSAS	304	1,021	29.8%	398	1,165	34.1%	14.6%	214.1%
MINNESOTA	790	2,366	33.4%	959	2,559	37.5%	12.2%	158.5%
MISSOURI	576	2,177	26.5%	1,024	2,827	36.2%	36.8%	569.7%
NEBRASKA	210	779	26.9%	262	868	30.2%	12.3%	205.9%
NORTH DAKOTA	134	471	28.6%	162	533	30.3%	6.1%	274.8%
SOUTH DAKOTA	122	511	23.8%	152	539	28.1%	18.0%	386.3%
Southeast:	*9,274*	*28,155*	*32.9%*	*12,511*	*32,483*	*38.5%*	*16.9%*	*333.7%*
ALABAMA	601	2,101	28.6%	800	2,347	34.1%	19.0%	258.6%
ARKANSAS	474	1,250	37.9%	568	1,439	39.5%	4.1%	251.5%
FLORIDA	1,427	4,576	31.2%	1,878	5,209	36.1%	15.7%	487.5%
GEORGIA	1,002	3,136	31.9%	1,252	3,553	35.2%	10.3%	192.5%
KENTUCKY	753	2,044	36.9%	1,077	2,493	43.2%	17.2%	460.6%
LOUISIANA	1,041	2,658	39.2%	1,532	3,249	47.1%	20.3%	435.2%
MISSISSIPPI	510	1,595	31.9%	660	1,822	36.2%	13.4%	251.0%
NORTH CAROLINA	1,020	2,942	34.7%	1,405	3,447	40.8%	17.6%	294.9%
SOUTH CAROLINA	642	1,892	33.9%	921	2,078	44.3%	30.5%	487.0%
TENNESSEE	970	2,717	35.7%	1,307	3,129	41.8%	17.0%	419.7%
VIRGINIA	548	2,237	24.5%	684	2,432	28.1%	14.9%	180.3%
WEST VIRGINIA	287	1,009	28.4%	428	1,284	33.3%	17.3%	755.4%
Southwest:	*3,090*	*11,035*	*28.0%*	*4,176*	*12,553*	*33.3%*	*18.8%*	*202.9%*
ARIZONA	408	1,619	25.2%	520	1,810	28.7%	13.9%	N/A
NEW MEXICO	213	959	22.2%	297	1,118	26.5%	19.6%	375.2%
OKLAHOMA	515	1,568	32.9%	642	1,788	35.9%	9.3%	138.2%
TEXAS	1,954	6,889	28.4%	2,717	7,837	34.7%	22.3%	169.0%
Rocky Mountain:	*831*	*3,996*	*20.8%*	*1,077*	*4,420*	*24.4%*	*17.1%*	*218.6%*
COLORADO	306	1,429	21.4%	423	1,707	24.8%	16.0%	147.3%
IDAHO	124	569	21.8%	161	590	27.3%	24.7%	305.9%
MONTANA	133	591	22.5%	172	687	25.0%	11.3%	340.6%
UTAH	224	838	26.8%	250	839	29.8%	11.4%	287.6%
WYOMING	44	568	7.7%	71	597	11.8%	52.8%	378.6%
Far West:	*5,017*	*18,651*	*26.9%*	*5,954*	*21,954*	*27.1%*	*0.8%*	*86.8%*
CALIFORNIA	3,870	13,932	27.8%	4,531	16,885	26.8%	-3.4%	61.4%
NEVADA	74	442	16.6%	106	544	19.6%	17.7%	240.8%
OREGON	369	1,708	21.6%	476	1,694	28.1%	29.9%	331.5%
WASHINGTON	704	2,568	27.4%	840	2,832	29.7%	8.2%	224.7%
ALASKA	89	717	12.5%	101	738	13.6%	9.4%	678.1%
HAWAII	121	598	20.3%	143	739	19.4%	-4.4%	170.3%
PUERTO RICO	81	3,082	2.6%	75	2,916	2.6%	-2.0%	-53.3%
TERRITORIES	7	514	1.3%	8	417	1.9%	38.9%	153.0%
TOTAL	*$40,857*	*$134,457*	*30.4%*	*$52,533*	*$153,350*	*34.3%* 0	*12.7%*	*171.1%*

Source: U.S. Treasury and Census publications. Totals differ slightly from OMB estimates.

Table 6. State and local government 1990 spending by function (dollars in millions).

	Total	Elem/Sec Education	Trans- portation	Public Welfare	Health & Hospitals	Public Safety	Percent Change from 1977 Total	El/Sec Educ	Trans- ortation	Publ Welf	Hlth & Hosp	S
U.S.	$834,818	$202,009	$70,628	$110,518	$74,635	$73,968	204.4%	182.3%	175.4%	207.8%	224.0%	25
CONNECTICUT	13,421	3,233	1,358	1,792	1,017	1,111	266.8%	206.6%	431.4%	308.8%	358.0%	27
MAINE	4,017	1,072	390	697	198	254	234.2%	230.7%	136.0%	296.8%	303.7%	26
MASSACHUSETTS	23,264	4,678	1,220	4,563	2,232	2,147	179.9%	105.3%	112.1%	208.1%	284.2%	20
NEW HAMPSHIRE	3,286	932	347	369	155	285	245.0%	292.8%	124.9%	222.9%	136.8%	34
RHODE ISLAND	3,685	809	286	550	258	324	213.0%	202.9%	330.7%	152.9%	169.1%	25
VERMONT	2,036	543	210	275	68	106	220.7%	254.3%	147.0%	225.3%	100.5%	21
DELAWARE	2,575	550	265	229	148	195	203.3%	168.9%	242.3%	206.1%	241.9%	24
DIST OF COL	4,020	573	126	672	443	824	169.0%	101.2%	138.0%	153.7%	274.2%	20
MARYLAND	16,633	3,961	1,690	1,901	808	1,704	181.5%	135.1%	218.4%	222.7%	93.1%	25
NEW JERSEY	29,938	7,726	2,045	3,637	1,561	2,613	203.2%	188.6%	209.4%	194.7%	183.2%	21
NEW YORK	90,332	19,733	5,907	16,002	9,254	8,585	186.1%	168.3%	227.3%	186.7%	221.1%	24
PENNSYLVANIA	35,696	10,050	3,089	5,222	1,941	2,271	156.8%	174.9%	149.6%	116.1%	95.8%	14
ILLINOIS	34,573	8,217	3,471	4,536	2,267	3,105	141.3%	117.4%	127.3%	117.8%	125.2%	16
INDIANA	15,310	4,121	1,162	1,998	1,587	1,036	203.0%	167.3%	121.5%	321.9%	228.0%	20
MICHIGAN	31,203	7,988	2,077	4,672	3,286	2,682	148.1%	136.0%	110.9%	127.8%	210.3%	18
OHIO	32,046	8,325	2,267	5,362	2,661	2,622	171.6%	136.6%	125.8%	305.5%	148.6%	20
WISCONSIN	16,720	4,281	1,465	2,695	1,061	1,309	168.8%	164.5%	125.6%	179.9%	144.2%	21
IOWA	8,842	2,082	1,034	1,215	954	477	148.9%	106.6%	94.5%	230.7%	231.5%	16
KANSAS	7,493	1,915	865	758	642	571	171.5%	164.5%	138.5%	155.4%	142.8%	28
MINNESOTA	17,122	4,016	1,799	2,561	1,503	936	195.8%	163.8%	179.5%	235.7%	235.1%	21
MISSOURI	12,489	3,658	1,235	1,439	1,181	1,022	175.9%	181.9%	127.4%	222.2%	162.0%	18
NEBRASKA	4,818	1,278	549	530	494	298	158.5%	133.6%	100.3%	275.4%	213.3%	18
NORTH DAKOTA	2,170	504	264	250	86	86	146.6%	141.0%	65.2%	269.8%	177.5%	14
SOUTH DAKOTA	1,948	500	287	196	112	111	137.7%	144.4%	102.4%	179.6%	100.9%	16
ALABAMA	10,868	2,338	982	1,073	1,810	719	188.5%	179.1%	99.8%	185.8%	250.0%	23
ARKANSAS	5,352	1,395	506	789	534	338	182.9%	190.5%	81.2%	230.6%	189.1%	23
FLORIDA	40,884	10,024	3,913	3,728	3,915	4,438	341.8%	309.5%	356.6%	663.4%	277.9%	37
GEORGIA	19,648	5,097	1,649	2,160	3,049	1,699	277.1%	271.9%	198.0%	318.4%	258.2%	37
KENTUCKY	9,606	1,999	919	1,432	706	653	171.3%	139.9%	91.7%	203.6%	235.4%	18
LOUISIANA	12,926	2,895	1,183	1,352	1,563	957	177.7%	171.6%	63.4%	204.7%	212.5%	13
MISSISSIPPI	6,593	1,589	584	711	1,047	389	169.9%	194.8%	51.3%	203.9%	258.1%	20
NORTH CAROLINA	18,715	4,924	1,694	1,919	2,266	1,502	240.8%	211.3%	219.2%	343.0%	292.4%	27
SOUTH CAROLINA	9,970	2,624	695	1,080	1,488	741	273.8%	270.9%	230.7%	348.7%	318.7%	31
TENNESSEE	12,704	2,664	1,397	1,384	1,598	1,074	198.5%	160.0%	173.8%	221.2%	238.4%	25
VIRGINIA	19,494	5,187	2,254	1,590	1,749	1,817	249.6%	244.1%	201.9%	215.5%	285.6%	32
WEST VIRGINIA	4,644	1,203	499	633	352	184	134.6%	119.0%	33.6%	237.0%	152.1%	11
ARIZONA	13,040	2,825	1,933	1,284	627	1,290	347.5%	224.4%	511.8%	898.5%	184.1%	40
NEW MEXICO	4,963	1,134	537	460	425	441	277.7%	167.4%	243.2%	323.9%	312.9%	35
OKLAHOMA	8,428	2,105	853	1,102	866	650	190.1%	175.8%	159.3%	205.7%	262.5%	24
TEXAS	47,230	13,939	4,798	4,304	4,115	4,045	262.4%	281.9%	275.0%	258.6%	212.4%	37
COLORADO	10,707	2,681	1,147	1,027	735	995	205.6%	160.8%	211.2%	218.3%	162.5%	30
IDAHO	2,651	647	343	250	240	205	170.1%	171.9%	114.9%	218.6%	216.5%	20
MONTANA	2,513	698	331	293	144	131	140.2%	139.0%	58.5%	263.3%	135.8%	14
UTAH	4,961	1,239	481	461	385	341	223.3%	163.1%	193.1%	282.1%	321.3%	27
WYOMING	2,158	542	293	109	232	133	232.5%	208.6%	151.6%	308.8%	271.6%	28
CALIFORNIA	112,945	24,161	6,269	17,127	10,006	13,134	237.5%	197.5%	239.5%	185.4%	308.9%	32
NEVADA	4,124	923	552	254	316	561	348.6%	337.4%	360.2%	325.5%	208.9%	44
OREGON	9,565	2,554	849	960	678	874	187.7%	183.4%	154.1%	172.6%	243.0%	23
WASHINGTON	16,613	4,280	1,405	2,099	1,355	1,396	229.7%	231.1%	120.1%	295.0%	355.5%	26
ALASKA	5,376	913	651	375	206	298	302.6%	173.1%	183.5%	553.2%	353.1%	24
HAWAII	4,414	685	503	440	310	292	156.9%	133.9%	124.1%	127.2%	191.9%	19

Source: U.S. Bureau of the Census; Government Finances.

Table 7. Change in shares of state and local government 1990 spending, 1977–1990.

	Share of Total 1990 Spending					Change in Share Since 1977				
	El/Sec Educ	Trans- Portation	Public Welfare	Health & Hospitals	Public Safety	El/Sec Educ	Trans- Portation	Public Welfare	Health & Hospitals	Public Safety
U.S.	24.2%	8.5%	13.2%	8.9%	8.9%	-1.9%	-0.9%	0.1%	0.5%	1.3%
CONNECTICUT	24.1%	10.1%	13.4%	7.6%	8.3%	-4.7%	3.1%	1.4%	1.5%	0.2%
MAINE	26.7%	9.7%	17.3%	4.9%	6.3%	-0.3%	-4.0%	2.7%	0.8%	0.5%
MASSACHUSETTS	20.1%	5.2%	19.6%	9.6%	9.2%	-7.3%	-1.7%	1.8%	2.6%	0.6%
NEW HAMPSHIRE	28.4%	10.6%	11.2%	4.7%	8.7%	3.5%	-5.6%	-0.8%	-2.2%	1.9%
RHODE ISLAND	22.0%	7.8%	14.9%	7.0%	8.8%	-0.7%	2.1%	-3.5%	-1.1%	1.0%
VERMONT	26.7%	10.3%	13.5%	3.4%	5.2%	2.5%	-3.1%	0.2%	-2.0%	-0.1%
DELAWARE	21.4%	10.3%	8.9%	5.7%	7.6%	-2.7%	1.2%	0.1%	0.6%	1.0%
DIST OF COL	14.3%	3.1%	16.7%	11.0%	20.5%	-4.8%	-0.4%	-1.0%	3.1%	2.1%
MARYLAND	23.8%	10.2%	11.4%	4.9%	10.2%	-4.7%	1.2%	1.5%	-2.2%	2.1%
NEW JERSEY	25.8%	6.8%	12.1%	5.2%	8.7%	-1.3%	0.1%	-0.4%	-0.4%	0.4%
NEW YORK	21.8%	6.5%	17.7%	10.2%	9.5%	-1.5%	0.8%	0.0%	1.1%	1.7%
PENNSYLVANIA	28.2%	8.7%	14.6%	5.4%	6.4%	1.9%	-0.3%	-2.8%	-1.7%	-0.2%
ILLINOIS	23.8%	10.0%	13.1%	6.6%	9.0%	-2.6%	-0.6%	-1.4%	-0.5%	0.7%
INDIANA	26.9%	7.6%	13.1%	10.4%	6.8%	-3.6%	-2.8%	3.7%	0.8%	0.1%
MICHIGAN	25.6%	6.7%	15.0%	10.5%	8.6%	-1.3%	-1.2%	-1.3%	2.1%	1.2%
OHIO	26.0%	7.1%	16.7%	8.3%	8.2%	-3.8%	-1.4%	5.5%	-0.8%	1.0%
WISCONSIN	25.6%	8.8%	16.1%	6.3%	7.8%	-0.4%	-1.7%	0.6%	-0.6%	1.2%
IOWA	23.5%	11.7%	13.7%	10.8%	5.4%	-4.8%	-3.3%	3.4%	2.7%	0.3%
KANSAS	25.6%	11.5%	10.1%	8.6%	7.6%	-0.7%	-1.6%	-0.6%	-1.0%	2.2%
MINNESOTA	23.5%	10.5%	15.0%	8.8%	5.5%	-2.9%	-0.6%	1.8%	1.0%	0.4%
MISSOURI	29.3%	9.9%	11.5%	9.5%	8.2%	0.6%	-2.1%	1.7%	-0.5%	0.2%
NEBRASKA	26.5%	11.4%	11.0%	10.3%	6.2%	-2.8%	-3.3%	3.4%	1.8%	0.6%
NORTH DAKOTA	23.2%	12.2%	11.5%	4.0%	4.0%	-0.5%	-6.0%	3.8%	0.4%	0.0%
SOUTH DAKOTA	25.7%	14.7%	10.1%	5.7%	5.7%	0.7%	-2.6%	1.5%	-1.1%	0.6%
ALABAMA	21.5%	9.0%	9.9%	16.7%	6.6%	-0.7%	-4.0%	-0.1%	2.9%	1.0%
ARKANSAS	26.1%	9.5%	14.7%	10.0%	6.3%	0.7%	-5.3%	2.1%	0.2%	1.1%
FLORIDA	24.5%	9.6%	9.1%	9.6%	10.9%	-1.9%	0.3%	3.8%	-1.6%	0.8%
GEORGIA	25.9%	8.4%	11.0%	15.5%	8.6%	-0.4%	-2.2%	1.1%	-0.8%	1.7%
KENTUCKY	20.8%	9.6%	14.9%	7.3%	6.8%	-2.7%	-4.0%	1.6%	1.4%	0.4%
LOUISIANA	22.4%	9.2%	10.5%	12.1%	7.4%	-0.5%	-6.4%	0.9%	1.3%	-1.2%
MISSISSIPPI	24.1%	8.9%	10.8%	15.9%	5.9%	2.0%	-7.0%	1.2%	3.9%	0.7%
NORTH CAROLINA	26.3%	9.0%	10.3%	12.1%	8.0%	-2.5%	-0.6%	2.4%	1.6%	0.7%
SOUTH CAROLINA	26.3%	7.0%	10.8%	14.9%	7.4%	-0.2%	-0.9%	1.8%	1.6%	0.8%
TENNESSEE	21.0%	11.0%	10.9%	12.6%	8.5%	-3.1%	-1.0%	0.8%	1.5%	1.4%
VIRGINIA	26.6%	11.6%	8.2%	9.0%	9.3%	-0.4%	-1.8%	-0.9%	0.8%	1.7%
WEST VIRGINIA	25.9%	10.8%	13.6%	7.6%	4.0%	-1.8%	-8.1%	4.1%	0.5%	-0.4%
ARIZONA	21.7%	14.8%	9.8%	4.8%	9.9%	-8.2%	4.0%	5.4%	-2.8%	1.2%
NEW MEXICO	22.9%	10.8%	9.3%	8.6%	8.9%	-7.7%	-0.5%	1.4%	1.1%	1.9%
OKLAHOMA	25.0%	10.1%	13.1%	10.3%	7.7%	-1.3%	-1.2%	0.7%	2.1%	1.2%
TEXAS	29.5%	10.2%	9.1%	8.7%	8.6%	1.5%	0.3%	-0.1%	-1.4%	2.0%
COLORADO	25.0%	10.7%	9.6%	6.9%	9.3%	-4.3%	0.2%	0.4%	-1.1%	2.3%
IDAHO	24.4%	12.9%	9.4%	9.0%	7.7%	0.2%	-3.3%	1.4%	1.3%	0.9%
MONTANA	27.8%	13.2%	11.6%	5.7%	5.2%	-0.1%	-6.8%	3.9%	-0.1%	0.1%
UTAH	25.0%	9.7%	9.3%	7.8%	6.9%	-5.7%	-1.0%	1.4%	1.8%	1.0%
WYOMING	25.1%	13.6%	5.1%	10.8%	6.2%	-1.9%	-4.4%	0.9%	1.1%	0.8%
CALIFORNIA	21.4%	5.6%	15.2%	8.9%	11.6%	-2.9%	0.0%	-2.8%	1.5%	2.3%
NEVADA	22.4%	13.4%	6.2%	7.7%	13.6%	-0.6%	0.3%	-0.3%	-3.5%	2.4%
OREGON	26.5%	8.8%	9.9%	7.0%	9.0%	-0.4%	-1.2%	-0.6%	1.1%	1.3%
WASHINGTON	25.8%	8.5%	12.6%	8.2%	8.4%	0.1%	-4.2%	2.1%	2.3%	0.8%
ALASKA	17.0%	12.1%	7.0%	3.8%	5.5%	-8.1%	-5.1%	2.7%	0.4%	-0.8%
HAWAII	15.5%	11.4%	10.0%	7.0%	6.6%	-1.5%	-1.7%	-1.3%	0.8%	0.8%

Source: U.S. Bureau of the Census; Government Finances.

Traditional services such as education or transportation (mainly roads) shrank in importance.

Regional differences in grants also can be seen in these tables. Most southern states experienced more substantial growth on the combination of public welfare and health and hospitals than the country as a whole, and spent larger shares of their budgets on these purposes.

Medicaid as a share of state government expenditures

Perhaps a better feel for state differences in Medicaid spending can be achieved by looking at Medicaid in the context of state government spending. Table 8 displays these data, as published by the National Conference of State Budget Officers (NASBO). Once again, states with relatively small Medicaid programs in 1987 show the fastest growth. NASBO has estimated that state governments will spend 14 percent of their 1992 budget on Medicaid, growing to 16 percent in the near future.

Medicaid as a share of personal income

An alternative measure of Medicaid spending is to compare it to total state personal income, as measured in the national income and product accounts (see Table 9). This comparison measures Medicaid as a share of state economic activity, abstracting from the different levels of government in states. A wide variance among states clearly exists. Medicaid constituted over 3 percent of 1990 personal income for New York and the District of Columbia (10), than 1 percent for Virginia, Arizona, Colorado, Nevada, and Hawaii. Again, states in the Southeast show the fastest growth, though shares in New England states are both high and fast growing.

A caveat

While the comparisons shown here are probably valid, comparisons should be treated with caution. States have generated substantial amounts of Medicaid grants in recent years through a variety of mechanisms that generate resources from health care providers (provider taxes, voluntary contributions, intergovernmental transfers). While much of those resources has gone to improved health care, much has also gone to generating federal grant revenues for state general funds. As such, measuring increased Medicaid spending could mean an increased or decreased state commitment of its own resources to the program.

THE DECLINING FISCAL POSTURE OF THE STATES (11)

The severe recession of the early 1980s placed a great deal of strain on state and local governments. According to the National Association of State Budget Officers (NASBO), year-end balances sank to 1.5 percent of expenditures in

1983 from 9 percent in 1979 and 1980 (12). State and local governments simultaneously raised taxes and restrained expenditure growth. As the economy expanded in 1984 and 1985, revenues from the tax increases tended to exceed projections, and state fiscal postures rapidly improved. By 1985, state balances were over 5 percent. While catch-up spending and adjustments to the 1986 federal tax reform reduced balances somewhat during 1986 and 1987, by 1988 end-of-year balances totaled 4.8 percent.

These overall shifts are reflected in Table 10, which presents data from the state and local government sector of the national income and product accounts (NIPA). These data should be interpreted cautiously, since expenditures include capital construction often financed through borrowing, and the "surplus" is usually negative. Nonetheless, the change in the size of the surplus is an important indicator of overall shifts in the sector.

The substantial construction of the 1950s and 1960s kept the state and local sectors in a relatively consistent deficit posture through 1972. At that point, the initial distribution of general revenue sharing funds created a substantial surplus and began an unsettled period that has continued to this day. Construction has declined in the 1970s and 1980s, and deficits increasingly reflect unsettled governmental fiscal conditions.

The anti-recession grant distributions of the late 1970s and the state-belt tightening of the middle 1980s produced two periods of surplus. Beginning in 1987, however, state and local governments as a group began a period of sharp fiscal decline. In each of these years, problems in one year have been exacerbated by efforts to "manage" the problem of the previous year by delaying spending or speeding up receipts. If these estimates are correct, state and local governments experienced a cumulative deficit of $125 billion in 1987–1991.

Despite tax increases in most states, NASBO reports that year-end state balances fell to 3.4 percent in 1990 and 1.8 percent in 1991. It should be noted that the NASBO data show a substantially better fiscal posture for states than the NIPA data show for the state and local sector as a whole. Local governments, stung by sharp cutbacks in federal aid and declining property tax revenues, turned to state governments for assistance, but with little success.

Table 11 displays the NASBO data for 1987 and 1991, estimates for 1992, and governors' budget requests for 1993. Overall, balances continue to drop in 1992 and 1993. The South, with the worst fiscal posture in 1987, shows substantial improvement in 1991 despite the fastest increase in expenditures. At the other extreme, the fiscal situation of the northeastern states as a group shows a dramatic decline despite overall expenditure restraint. The western states continue with the healthiest overall fiscal posture, though with balances still half that of 1987.

The states thus entered the 1990s having, on net, raised tax rates, but with declining fiscal balances. Local governments were clamoring for aid. Discretionary grants-in-aid from Washington had been cut back. Given federal budget rules, and the immense amounts of money being spent on

Table 8. Medicaid spending as a share of total state spending (state fiscal years; dollars in millions).

| | 1987 State Spending | | 1990 State Spending | | Share of Total Spending | | |
	Medicaid	Total	Medicaid	Total	1987	1990	% Change
U.S.	$41,506	$408,486	$62,359	$501,193	10.2%	12.4%	22.5%
CONNECTICUT	600	6,984	964	9,446	8.6%	10.2%	18.8%
MAINE	283	1,933	396	2,651	14.6%	14.9%	2.0%
MASSACHUSETTS	1,423	14,718	2,612	17,196	9.7%	15.2%	57.1%
NEW HAMPSHIRE	144	1,129	215	1,392	12.8%	15.4%	21.1%
RHODE ISLAND	293	1,640	428	2,246	17.9%	19.1%	6.7%
VERMONT	98	943	146	1,223	10.4%	11.9%	14.9%
DELAWARE	90	1,673	131	2,203	5.4%	5.9%	10.5%
DIST OF COL	298	3,210	N/A	N/A	9.3%	N/A	N/A
MARYLAND	804	8,700	1,152	11,312	9.2%	10.2%	10.2%
NEW JERSEY	1,551	13,247	2,256	16,408	11.7%	13.7%	17.4%
NEW YORK	6,330	36,018	8,362	46,361	17.6%	18.0%	2.6%
PENNSYLVANIA	2,125	18,130	2,670	21,814	11.7%	12.2%	4.4%
ILLINOIS	1,784	16,898	2,250	18,845	10.6%	11.9%	13.1%
INDIANA	933	7,376	1,446	9,011	12.6%	16.0%	26.9%
MICHIGAN	1,576	14,750	2,799	17,511	10.7%	16.0%	49.6%
OHIO	2,037	17,747	2,800	21,105	11.5%	13.3%	15.6%
WISCONSIN	1,114	10,902	1,423	11,019	10.2%	12.9%	26.4%
IOWA	428	6,646	624	7,001	6.4%	8.9%	38.4%
KANSAS	249	3,629	409	4,761	6.9%	8.6%	25.2%
MINNESOTA	1,109	10,011	1,421	9,986	11.1%	14.2%	28.5%
MISSOURI	566	6,452	832	8,020	8.8%	10.4%	18.3%
NEBRASKA	195	2,032	311	2,750	9.6%	11.3%	17.8%
NORTH DAKOTA	166	1,224	174	1,519	13.6%	11.5%	-15.5%
SOUTH DAKOTA	114	1,059	160	1,162	10.8%	13.8%	27.9%
ALABAMA	421	5,430	834	7,383	7.8%	11.3%	45.7%
ARKANSAS	358	3,486	600	4,555	10.3%	13.2%	28.3%
FLORIDA	1,394	16,888	2,407	22,812	8.3%	10.6%	27.8%
GEORGIA	911	7,900	1,497	11,817	11.5%	12.7%	9.9%
KENTUCKY	620	6,554	946	7,740	9.5%	12.2%	29.2%
LOUISIANA	882	7,381	1,319	8,483	11.9%	15.5%	30.1%
MISSISSIPPI	384	3,653	608	4,082	10.5%	14.9%	41.7%
NORTH CAROLINA	823	8,863	1,358	11,765	9.3%	11.5%	24.3%
SOUTH CAROLINA	421	5,437	752	7,683	7.7%	9.8%	26.4%
TENNESSEE	820	6,122	1,370	7,549	13.4%	18.1%	35.5%
VIRGINIA	702	9,406	1,004	12,298	7.5%	8.2%	9.4%
WEST VIRGINIA	255	3,355	451	3,680	7.6%	12.3%	61.2%
ARIZONA	N/A	4,259	643	5,985	N/A	10.7%	N/A
NEW MEXICO	192	2,694	279	3,834	7.1%	7.3%	2.1%
OKLAHOMA	525	5,054	706	5,920	10.4%	11.9%	14.8%
TEXAS	824	17,757	3,069	23,531	4.6%	13.0%	181.1%
COLORADO	399	4,476	584	5,292	8.9%	11.0%	23.8%
IDAHO	84	1,333	149	1,815	6.3%	8.2%	30.3%
MONTANA	144	1,537	172	1,764	9.4%	9.8%	4.1%
UTAH	208	2,683	270	3,212	7.8%	8.4%	8.4%
WYOMING	41	1,726	61	1,366	2.4%	4.5%	88.0%
CALIFORNIA	5,329	52,825	7,170	67,247	10.1%	10.7%	5.7%
NEVADA	121	1,368	N/A	N/A	8.8%	N/A	N/A
OREGON	286	5,982	524	6,987	4.8%	7.5%	56.9%
WASHINGTON	795	8,902	1,209	11,350	8.9%	10.7%	19.3%
ALASKA	75	3,348	156	3,726	2.2%	4.2%	86.9%
HAWAII	176	3,022	239	4,375	5.8%	5.5%	-6.2%

Source: State Expenditure Survey; National Association of State Fiscal Officers.

Table 9. Medicaid as a share of personal income, 1986–1990.

	1986	1989	1990	Percent Change 1986-90	Percent Change 1989-90
U.S.	1.24%	1.39%	1.57%	26.6%	12.8%
CONNECTICUT	1.14%	1.35%	1.58%	38.4%	17.1%
MAINE	1.80%	1.87%	2.21%	22.7%	18.2%
MASSACHUSETTS	1.62%	2.16%	2.48%	53.2%	14.9%
NEW HAMPSHIRE	0.82%	0.88%	1.04%	27.0%	18.6%
RHODE ISLAND	1.99%	2.12%	2.40%	20.7%	13.3%
VERMONT	1.30%	1.40%	1.66%	27.2%	18.5%
DELAWARE	0.86%	0.95%	1.02%	18.8%	7.1%
DIST OF COLUMBIA	2.79%	2.71%	3.05%	9.6%	12.6%
MARYLAND	1.01%	1.05%	1.20%	18.8%	14.5%
NEW JERSEY	0.95%	1.14%	1.27%	32.7%	10.8%
NEW YORK	2.84%	2.94%	3.21%	12.9%	9.3%
PENNSYLVANIA	1.29%	1.36%	1.40%	9.0%	3.0%
ILLINOIS	0.96%	1.00%	1.05%	10.2%	4.9%
INDIANA	1.28%	1.41%	1.67%	30.3%	18.6%
MICHIGAN	1.36%	1.43%	1.55%	14.2%	8.4%
OHIO	1.43%	1.59%	1.78%	24.4%	12.3%
WISCONSIN	1.60%	1.64%	1.80%	12.5%	9.9%
IOWA	1.02%	1.25%	1.42%	38.8%	13.7%
KANSAS	0.79%	0.97%	1.14%	44.8%	17.9%
MINNESOTA	1.70%	1.73%	1.90%	12.0%	10.0%
MISSOURI	0.88%	1.02%	1.12%	28.0%	9.6%
NEBRASKA	0.93%	1.10%	1.24%	33.6%	13.1%
NORTH DAKOTA	2.11%	2.01%	2.13%	1.0%	5.6%
SOUTH DAKOTA	1.29%	1.53%	1.60%	23.6%	4.5%
ALABAMA	0.93%	1.05%	1.58%	68.6%	49.9%
ARKANSAS	1.62%	1.74%	1.92%	18.1%	10.5%
FLORIDA	0.64%	0.94%	1.13%	76.7%	20.7%
GEORGIA	1.05%	1.29%	1.50%	43.2%	16.9%
KENTUCKY	1.38%	1.71%	1.94%	40.8%	14.0%
LOUISIANA	1.64%	2.05%	2.45%	50.0%	19.9%
MISSISSIPPI	1.36%	1.70%	2.01%	48.6%	18.4%
NORTH CAROLINA	1.00%	1.24%	1.45%	44.2%	16.5%
SOUTH CAROLINA	1.13%	1.31%	1.86%	65.6%	42.9%
TENNESSEE	1.36%	1.64%	1.99%	46.2%	20.8%
VIRGINIA	0.72%	0.77%	0.90%	26.2%	17.1%
WEST VIRGINIA	1.30%	1.65%	1.74%	33.7%	5.4%
ARIZONA	0.25%	0.80%	0.97%	283.8%	20.4%
NEW MEXICO	1.05%	1.27%	1.43%	37.0%	12.9%
OKLAHOMA	1.22%	1.49%	1.55%	27.4%	4.3%
TEXAS	0.75%	0.93%	1.18%	57.6%	26.8%
COLORADO	0.71%	0.89%	0.94%	32.3%	6.0%
IDAHO	0.75%	0.95%	1.09%	45.2%	14.2%
MONTANA	1.31%	1.53%	1.69%	28.5%	9.9%
UTAH	0.99%	1.00%	1.22%	23.3%	22.7%
WYOMING	0.54%	0.80%	1.07%	98.0%	33.2%
CALIFORNIA	1.04%	1.07%	1.17%	12.3%	9.3%
NEVADA	0.56%	0.56%	0.71%	28.5%	28.7%
OREGON	0.80%	1.00%	1.16%	44.0%	15.4%
WASHINGTON	1.04%	1.25%	1.42%	35.9%	13.2%
ALASKA	0.89%	1.23%	1.36%	53.2%	10.6%
HAWAII	0.93%	0.93%	0.95%	1.9%	2.6%

Source: National Income Products Accounts

Table 10. State and local government summary finances, 1958–1991
(calendar years; dollars in millions).

Year	Receipts	Expend	Surplus	Surplus as % of Receipts	Grants Amount	% of Receipts
1958	37,398	41,589	-4,191	-11.2%	5,641	15.1%
1959	41,319	43,788	-2,469	-6.0%	6,848	16.6%
1960	44,181	46,420	-2,239	-5.1%	6,526	14.8%
1961	47,829	50,651	-2,822	-5.9%	7,245	15.1%
1962	51,736	53,862	-2,126	-4.1%	7,979	15.4%
1963	55,804	58,162	-2,358	-4.2%	9,141	16.4%
1964	61,153	63,353	-2,200	-3.6%	10,433	17.1%
1965	65,961	69,407	-3,446	-5.2%	11,121	16.9%
1966	74,227	77,712	-3,485	-4.7%	14,384	19.4%
1967	81,194	87,064	-5,870	-7.2%	15,912	19.6%
1968	93,371	98,555	-5,184	-5.6%	18,587	19.9%
1969	104,358	108,713	-4,355	-4.2%	20,346	19.5%
1970	116,832	121,926	-5,094	-4.4%	24,447	20.9%
1971	131,811	136,895	-5,084	-3.9%	29,011	22.0%
1972	154,109	149,349	4,760	3.1%	37,528	24.4%
1973	167,855	164,031	3,824	2.3%	40,563	24.2%
1974	180,851	184,660	-3,809	-2.1%	43,940	24.3%
1975	202,432	210,918	-8,486	-4.2%	54,558	27.0%
1976	226,550	227,573	-1,023	-0.5%	61,101	27.0%
1977	250,988	243,335	7,653	3.0%	67,536	26.9%
1978	274,392	263,508	10,884	4.0%	77,261	28.2%
1979	290,430	288,987	1,443	0.5%	80,510	27.7%
1980	315,913	318,070	-2,157	-0.7%	88,678	28.1%
1981	339,790	341,148	-1,358	-0.4%	87,893	25.9%
1982	348,292	358,002	-9,710	-2.8%	83,856	24.1%
1983	376,149	377,432	-1,283	-0.3%	86,979	23.1%
1984	420,068	404,852	15,216	3.6%	94,386	22.5%
1985	449,571	440,386	9,185	2.0%	100,275	22.3%
1986	482,380	480,844	1,536	0.3%	107,637	22.3%
1987	499,520	514,224	-14,704	-2.9%	102,847	20.6%
1988	530,937	549,339	-18,402	-3.5%	111,262	21.0%
1989	569,408	588,624	-19,216	-3.4%	118,222	20.8%
1990	609,827	647,884	-38,057	-6.2%	132,201	21.7%
1991	651,245	686,554	-35,309	-5.4%	152,827	23.5%

Note: This table displays state and local government receipts and expenditures, excluding the operations of social insurance funds, as represented in the National Income Product Accounts.

Table 11. State government expenditure growth and fiscal margins, 1987–1993 (state fiscal years).

	Balances as Percent of Expenditures				Percent Growth in Expenditures		
	1987	1991	1992 est.	1993 est.	1987-91	1991-92 est.	1992-93 est.
CONNECTICUT	0.0	-14.6	0.0	0.0	51.4	5.0	4.5
MAINE	5.7	0.3	0.0	0.0	51.3	-4.0	3.0
MASSACHUSETTS	0.4	1.7	0.9	0.6	28.0	-0.4	3.1
NEW HAMPSHIRE	4.5	-3.8	-0.6	0.2	25.3	9.3	4.8
RHODE ISLAND	9.7	0.2	0.5	1.7	29.2	20.8	-18.2
VERMONT	13.8	-8.9	-7.7	-1.9	53.1	2.5	0.2
DELAWARE	18.3	9.4	8.7	8.1	30.3	2.1	-0.4
DIST OF COLUMBIA	N/A	N/A	N/A	N/A	N/A	N/A	N/A
MARYLAND	4.7	0.0	0.2	1.5	39.7	-1.0	10.2
NEW JERSEY	7.9	0.0	2.8	1.5	33.4	19.5	4.6
NEW YORK	0.7	0.0	0.0	0.2	23.2	3.2	1.4
PENNSYLVANIA	3.6	-3.6	0.0	0.0	28.3	9.8	4.2
ILLINOIS	1.5	0.9	0.9	1.7	11.2	4.3	0.5
INDIANA	3.1	7.4	6.5	2.8	77.9	-0.8	8.1
MICHIGAN	0.2	0.2	-7.5	2.6	20.3	1.5	1.1
OHIO	2.1	3.4	-0.1	-3.7	20.7	4.3	7.2
WISCONSIN	4.6	1.8	1.8	1.1	25.5	3.5	5.1
IOWA	0.0	0.0	0.5	0.3	43.0	2.3	4.4
KANSAS	4.2	6.5	5.0	6.7	44.5	0.0	1.2
MINNESOTA	9.3	8.0	3.9	4.1	33.6	-5.9	-1.5
MISSOURI	1.5	0.9	1.1	2.0	29.6	2.2	3.5
NEBRASKA	6.5	14.1	10.9	8.0	72.0	5.1	3.0
NORTH DAKOTA	4.4	24.3	15.3	7.7	-3.9	12.2	4.3
SOUTH DAKOTA	9.8	2.1	3.5	4.2	42.5	9.0	4.7
ALABAMA	2.7	0.0	0.0	0.0	28.7	-1.4	3.9
ARKANSAS	0.0	0.0	0.0	0.0	12.4	2.6	7.5
FLORIDA	0.5	1.3	0.6	1.5	41.7	1.7	16.5
GEORGIA	2.8	0.5	0.0	0.0	37.4	1.1	9.1
KENTUCKY	5.7	4.5	1.1	1.0	43.7	10.1	0.1
LOUISIANA	-11.7	9.2	0.0	0.0	18.8	-1.2	2.7
MISSISSIPPI	7.7	2.4	2.2	3.6	29.0	-0.9	0.7
NORTH CAROLINA	6.8	0.0	1.3	5.1	41.4	4.2	3.6
SOUTH CAROLINA	3.4	1.8	1.8	2.6	29.7	-2.2	5.9
TENNESSEE	0.7	0.2	0.4	1.0	30.9	-0.1	0.8
VIRGINIA	3.0	0.0	0.4	0.0	36.0	-1.1	0.8
WEST VIRGINIA	2.0	4.7	1.2	0.0	17.2	5.1	4.6
ARIZONA	2.3	1.3	0.1	0.7	38.7	5.3	2.7
NEW MEXICO	8.0	4.1	3.5	3.6	31.8	7.6	1.8
OKLAHOMA	0.0	12.4	12.6	12.5	49.0	3.8	4.4
TEXAS	-9.9	4.7	-1.5	1.0	56.7	12.6	5.1
COLORADO	2.2	0.6	2.7	-2.2	29.9	4.1	11.0
IDAHO	0.0	7.5	2.6	2.6	51.1	8.7	1.9
MONTANA	2.6	13.1	3.1	0.8	15.1	15.6	1.7
UTAH	2.3	5.2	4.5	3.3	36.2	6.3	4.2
WYOMING	11.6	11.1	9.6	-7.9	9.9	-9.4	6.9
CALIFORNIA	2.0	-3.1	-3.1	1.2	27.9	8.6	0.2
NEVADA	4.7	6.8	4.3	4.9	61.1	7.9	3.6
OREGON	12.8	16.1	10.8	5.9	35.5	13.7	8.3
WASHINGTON	0.2	10.4	2.1	1.0	44.0	9.2	0.2
ALASKA	0.8	56.4	28.1	-21.2	15.5	3.3	-4.3
HAWAII	20.0	12.4	13.8	2.4	65.4	-1.1	19.0
U.S.	2.6	0.9	0.4	1.3	30.0	5.1	3.4

Sources: National Association of State Budget Officers; Fiscal Survey of the States; various years.

the savings and loan industry, these grants could not be expected to grow despite need. Major new requirements had been placed on the states, particularly for Medicaid, as new mandates originating in Congressman Henry Waxman's Health and Environment Subcommittee were being enacted annually. By the summer of 1990, 49 governors of all political persuasions voted for a National Governors' Association resolution requesting both no new mandates and a delay in those already enacted.

The new Medicaid requirements, which often mandated eligibility based on income, hit southern states particularly hard. These states generally had smaller Medicaid benefit packages, less intrusive state oversight of providers, less expansive AFDC and SSI eligibility, and a higher share of families with incomes under the poverty line. The new mandates therefore required greater expansions in virtually all Medicaid cost areas—benefits, administration, and eligibility.

In addition to the mandates, though, many states were desirous of expanding their Medicaid programs in certain areas. For example, the Southern Governors' Association in 1985 adopted a policy encouraging states to expand their programs for pregnant women and children. In 1986, SGA began a campaign that eventually led to the federal government's decoupling Medicaid eligibility from AFDC eligibility for this purpose. Similarly, many states recognized the need to provide additional Medicaid payments to hospitals with disproportionate shares (DSH) of Medicaid and uncompensated care.

Table 12 shows the growth in federal Medicaid grants from 1986–1990, and projections to 1993, with states grouped into three broad regions. Grants to southern states grew 91 percent over this period, as compared to 71 percent for western states and only 50 percent for the Northeast. Projected 1993 Medicaid growth in southern states continues to significantly outstrip that of the rest of the country.

ONE SOLUTION—INCREASED FEDERAL MEDICAID MATCHING

Fortunately for most states, the federal share of Medicaid benefit costs was increasing. That share, the federal medical assistance percentage (FMAP), changes every year and is based on a state's per capita personal income relative to the country as a whole. A state with precisely average per capita income receives a 55.00 percent FMAP. Mississippi has the highest 1992 FMAP (79.99 percent), and 11 states and the District of Columbia received the statutory minimum of 50.00 percent.

Through the 1970s, state per capita incomes tended to converge on the national average. As a result, the average FMAP declined substantially. Incomes diverged in the 1980s, and FMAPs consequently grew.

Table 13 shows the change in FMAPs between 1986 and 1992 and the financial impact on different states. All western states not at the minimum and half the states in the other regions received substantial FMAP increases.

Most of the 11 states that experienced a reduction were on the East Coast. If the 1986 FMAPs had been in place in 1992, federal grants would have been $1.5 billion lower.

FMAPs will decline for most states in 1993 for two reasons. First, per capita incomes have begun to converge again. Second, the 1990 census counted substantially more people in California, effectively reducing the state's *measured* per capita income. California receives the minimum FMAP and was not affected. However, most other states looked wealthier relative to the national average and will experience a 1993 FMAP decline. FMAPs can now be estimated for 1994, and they are expected to continue to decline (13).

The increased FMAPs experienced by most states in the 1986–1992 period allowed them to partially finance their Medicaid expansions from increased federal reimbursements. At an extreme, Wyoming received a 1986–1992 Medicaid grant increase of $70 million, $23 million of which reflected the FMAP shift alone.

ANOTHER SOLUTION—INCREASED STATE LEVERAGE

As states began to expand their Medicaid programs dramatically, some recognized the value of increasing federal Medicaid reimbursement by innovative financing mechanisms under state control—donations and provider-specific taxes. With these mechanisms, health providers either voluntarily donate funds or are taxed to provide funds to the state Medicaid program. This permits the state to generate federal matching funds, returning substantially more to the program than originally paid through donations or taxes. Additionally, health services once financed entirely by state or local governments could direct funding through the state's Medicaid program through intergovernmental transfers, These three mechanisms could be used to generate funds to expand a state's Medicaid program, to share its costs among different types of health providers, or simply to increase provider reimbursements without involving state broad-based tax revenues.

Table 14 compares the sum of these devices (as reported to HCFA in February 1992) to the change in state Medicaid shares. For states such as Wyoming and Texas, the increase in state share already had been muted by the FMAP shift. Of the remaining state share requiring financing, states such as Alabama were able to provide virtually all the balance through devices. Alabama's federal Medicaid grant increased over $750 million between 1986 and 1992 (Table 12), and Alabama only had to provide $3.3 million from sources such as broad based taxes.

February data indicates that almost $7 billion of these financing mechanisms is being used to generate an estimate $10.7 billion in 1992 federal Medicaid grants. An estimated three eighths of the 1991–1992 increase in "state shares" was produced by these devices. At one extreme, New Hampshire's *increase* in Medicaid grants during federal fiscal year 1992 represented eight percent of two years' budgets, permitting the state to

Table 12. Growth in federal Medicaid grants by state and region, 1986–1993 (federal fiscal years; dollars in thousands).

STATE	1986	1990	1992	1993	Percent Change 1986-90	1990-92	1992-93
Alabama	$316,681	$601,096	$1,103,208	$1,157,228	89.8%	83.5%	4.9%
Arkansas	319,691	473,879	657,359	694,229	48.2%	38.7%	5.6%
Florida	612,055	1,426,640	2,284,667	2,956,960	133.1%	60.1%	29.4%
Georgia	591,612	1,001,648	1,677,578	2,075,942	69.3%	67.5%	23.7%
Kentucky	404,724	753,489	1,408,316	1,628,030	86.2%	86.9%	15.6%
Louisiana	527,468	1,041,136	2,295,300	2,332,139	97.4%	120.5%	1.6%
Mississippi	271,775	509,563	945,371	1,027,555	87.5%	85.5%	8.7%
North Carolina	546,785	1,020,188	1,722,422	1,761,315	86.6%	68.8%	2.3%
South Carolina	316,550	642,150	1,173,269	1,214,198	102.9%	82.7%	3.5%
Tennessee	551,921	970,166	1,684,482	1,926,260	75.8%	73.6%	14.4%
Texas	901,011	1,953,574	4,036,606	4,544,335	116.8%	106.6%	12.6%
Virginia	353,522	547,582	854,934	957,073	54.9%	56.1%	11.9%
West Virginia	169,806	286,527	790,926	849,900	68.7%	176.0%	7.5%
Connecticut	339,205	613,473	1,284,985	1,407,791	80.9%	109.5%	9.6%
Delaware	42,278	68,094	122,162	142,396	61.1%	79.4%	16.6%
District of Columbia	186,837	216,824	289,616	285,689	16.0%	33.6%	-1.4%
Illinois	922,096	1,276,352	2,276,195	2,537,504	38.4%	78.3%	11.5%
Indiana	570,564	945,091	1,417,609	1,519,125	65.6%	50.0%	7.2%
Maine	189,931	283,081	450,903	478,116	49.0%	59.3%	6.0%
Maryland	378,587	619,830	1,108,292	1,278,528	63.7%	78.8%	15.4%
Massachusetts	869,438	1,569,596	2,047,168	1,962,151	80.5%	30.4%	-4.2%
Michigan	1,059,468	1,506,062	2,197,966	2,399,846	42.2%	45.9%	9.2%
Minnesota	579,726	790,003	1,118,407	1,185,029	36.3%	41.6%	6.0%
New Hampshire	74,834	121,431	555,220	187,126	62.3%	357.2%	-66.3%
New Jersey	700,298	1,261,356	2,650,755	2,731,275	80.1%	110.2%	3.0%
New York	4,383,745	6,301,091	10,305,457	11,274,329	43.7%	63.6%	9.4%
Ohio	1,262,672	1,956,626	3,317,439	3,606,602	55.0%	69.5%	8.7%
Pennsylvania	1,285,746	1,813,671	3,517,196	3,192,168	41.1%	93.9%	-9.2%
Rhode Island	150,676	245,677	388,428	433,305	63.0%	58.1%	11.6%
Vermont	68,623	105,035	153,466	159,283	53.1%	46.1%	3.8%
Wisconsin	622,503	893,091	1,232,871	1,343,298	43.5%	38.0%	9.0%
Alaska	48,558	89,310	112,602	117,356	83.9%	26.1%	4.2%
Arizona	70,249	408,302	843,887	1,076,154	481.2%	106.7%	27.5%
California	2,552,537	3,869,906	6,596,454	6,782,361	51.6%	70.5%	2.8%
Colorado	177,117	305,526	534,422	550,353	72.5%	74.9%	3.0%
Hawaii	76,615	121,441	168,869	161,939	58.5%	39.1%	-4.1%
Idaho	60,936	124,383	205,602	234,374	104.1%	65.3%	14.0%
Iowa	235,498	414,143	619,093	670,053	75.9%	49.5%	8.2%
Kansas	145,048	304,195	600,572	684,302	109.7%	97.4%	13.9%
Missouri	356,309	576,412	1,137,824	896,894	61.8%	97.4%	-21.2%
Montana	86,205	132,755	205,865	247,237	54.0%	55.1%	20.1%
Nebraska	119,591	209,523	308,200	331,833	75.2%	47.1%	7.7%
Nevada	44,528	73,602	211,432	241,954	65.3%	187.3%	14.4%
New Mexico	122,860	212,842	394,488	436,569	73.2%	85.3%	10.7%
North Dakota	73,852	134,483	181,123	190,901	82.1%	34.7%	5.4%
Oklahoma	303,444	515,015	777,788	826,122	69.7%	51.0%	6.2%
Oregon	188,684	369,171	549,967	593,069	95.7%	49.0%	7.8%
South Dakota	75,080	121,809	179,139	196,511	62.2%	47.1%	9.7%
Utah	139,803	224,471	314,761	383,326	60.6%	40.2%	21.8%
Washington	354,649	703,965	1,129,907	1,259,648	98.5%	60.5%	11.5%
Wyoming	18,328	43,928	87,935	95,230	139.7%	100.2%	8.3%
South	5,883,601	11,227,638	20,634,438	23,125,164	90.8%	83.8%	12.1%
Northeast	13,687,227	20,586,384	34,434,135	36,123,561	50.4%	67.3%	4.9%
West	5,249,891	8,955,182	15,159,930	15,976,186	70.6%	69.3%	5.4%
U.S.	$24,820,719	$40,769,204	$70,228,503	$75,224,911	64.3%	72.3%	7.1%

Original source: U.S. Bureau of the Census, Federal Expenditures by State (1986,1990); HCFA form 25 submitted Feb. 1992 (1992,1993).

Table 13. Shifts in Medicaid matching rates by state and region, 1986–1994 (federal fiscal years; dollars in thousands).

STATE	Federal Share		Change, 1986-1992		Federal Share		Change, 1992-1994	
	1986	1992	% Change	Impact	1993	1994*	% Change	Impact
Texas	53.56 %	64.18 %	19.8%	$648,009	64.44 %	63.93 %	-0.4%	-$17,090
Louisiana	63.81	75.44	18.2%	348,936	73.71	72.99	-3.2%	-76,148
West Virginia	71.53	77.68	8.6%	61,825	76.29	75.85	-2.4%	-20,137
Kentucky	70.23	72.82	3.7%	49,074	71.69	71.02	-2.5%	-40,200
Arkansas	73.83	75.66	2.5%	15,434	74.41	73.97	-2.2%	-15,315
Mississippi	78.42	79.99	2.0%	18,147	79.01	78.64	-1.7%	-17,088
Alabama	72.30	72.93	0.9%	9,319	71.45	70.93	-2.7%	-31,663
Georgia	66.05	61.78	-6.5%	-111,348	62.08	62.57	1.3%	25,472
Virginia	53.14	50.00	-5.9%	-51,210	50.00	50.00	0.0%	0
North Carolina	69.18	66.52	-3.8%	-66,925	65.92	65.90	-0.9%	-16,088
Florida	56.16	54.69	-2.6%	-59,325	55.03	55.40	1.3%	36,823
Tennessee	70.20	68.41	-2.5%	-43,195	67.57	67.47	-1.4%	-26,320
South Carolina	72.70	72.66	-0.1%	-627	71.28	71.05	-2.2%	-26,599
Wisconsin	57.54	60.38	4.9%	56,229	60.42	59.97	-0.7%	-8,832
Ohio	58.30	60.63	4.0%	124,170	60.25	60.32	-0.5%	-18,078
Minnesota	53.41	54.43	1.9%	19,889	54.93	54.72	0.5%	5,951
Indiana	62.82	63.85	1.6%	22,473	63.21	63.11	-1.2%	-17,463
Pennsylvania	56.72	56.84	0.2%	7,197	55.48	55.16	-3.0%	-93,349
Delaware	50.00	50.12	0.2%	273	50.00	50.00	-0.2%	-325
Connecticut	50.00	50.00	0.0%	0	50.00	50.00	0.0%	0
District of Columbia	50.00	50.00	0.0%	0	50.00	50.00	0.0%	0
Illinois	50.00	50.00	0.0%	0	50.00	50.00	0.0%	0
Maryland	50.00	50.00	0.0%	0	50.00	50.00	0.0%	0
Massachusetts	50.00	50.00	0.0%	0	50.00	50.00	0.0%	0
New Jersey	50.00	50.00	0.0%	0	50.00	50.00	0.0%	0
New York	50.00	50.00	0.0%	0	50.00	50.00	0.0%	0
Michigan	56.79	55.41	-2.4%	-52,278	55.84	56.30	1.6%	36,707
Rhode Island	56.33	53.29	-5.4%	-21,676	53.64	54.64	2.5%	10,636
Vermont	67.06	61.37	-8.5%	-13,404	59.88	60.29	-1.8%	-2,707
New Hampshire	54.92	50.00	-9.0%	-53,923	50.00	50.00	0.0%	0
Maine	68.86	62.40	-9.4%	-45,218	61.81	62.11	-0.5%	-2,169
Wyoming	50.00	69.10	38.2%	23,435	67.11	65.91	-4.6%	-4,369
North Dakota	55.12	72.75	32.0%	42,401	72.21	69.69	-4.2%	-7,831
Oklahoma	57.60	70.74	22.8%	136,173	69.67	69.40	-1.9%	-15,026
Kansas	50.00	59.23	18.5%	91,255	58.18	58.09	-1.9%	-13,109
Nebraska	57.11	64.50	12.9%	33,607	61.32	60.94	-5.5%	-18,374
Iowa	58.90	65.04	10.4%	56,444	62.74	61.85	-4.9%	-32,818
Washington	50.06	54.98	9.8%	96,585	55.02	54.20	-1.4%	-17,115
Colorado	50.00	54.79	9.6%	44,711	54.42	54.02	-1.4%	-7,435
Montana	66.38	71.70	8.0%	14,858	70.92	69.28	-3.4%	-8,216
New Mexico	68.94	74.33	7.8%	27,677	73.85	73.57	-1.0%	-4,368
South Dakota	67.82	72.59	7.0%	11,535	70.27	68.06	-6.2%	-12,435
Idaho	69.39	73.24	5.5%	10,259	71.20	70.53	-3.7%	-8,473
Utah	72.62	75.11	3.4%	10,015	75.29	74.77	-0.5%	-1,662
Oregon	61.54	63.55	3.3%	15,870	62.39	61.98	-2.5%	-13,992
Hawaii	51.00	52.57	3.1%	4,749	50.00	50.00	-4.9%	-7,819
Arizona	62.28	62.61	0.5%	4,239	65.89	66.68	6.5%	63,589
Missouri	60.62	60.84	0.4%	4,000	60.26	60.51	-0.5%	-4,728
Alaska	50.00	50.00	0.0%	0	50.00	50.00	0.0%	0
California	50.00	50.00	0.0%	0	50.00	50.00	0.0%	0
Nevada	50.00	50.00	0.0%	0	52.28	53.22	6.4%	14,115
South	-----	-----	-----	818,114	-----	-----	-----	-224,352
Northeast	-----	-----	-----	43,734	-----	-----	-----	-89,627
West	-----	-----	-----	627,814	-----	-----	-----	-100,065
U.S.	-----	-----	-----	$1,489,661	-----	-----	-----	-$414,044

*Estimates based on preliminary personal income data. Final data will become available in August 1992

Table 14. Sources of financing for 1986–1992 changes in the state share of Medicaid (federal fiscal years; dollars in thousands).

STATE	State Share		Change, 1986-1992		Financing of Change in State Share		
	1986	1992	Amount	Percent	Change from 1986 FMAP	Total Devices	Other Sources
Alabama	$122,664	$413,995	$291,331	237.5%	$9,319	$288,005	$3,326
Arkansas	112,034	219,351	107,317	95.8%	15,434	27,737	79,580
Florida	466,680	1,893,044	1,426,364	305.6%	-59,325	276,200	1,150,164
Georgia	294,482	1,041,735	747,253	253.8%	-111,348	104,966	642,287
Kentucky	175,827	518,064	342,237	194.6%	49,074	162,083	180,154
Louisiana	303,044	776,756	473,712	156.3%	348,936	222,635	251,077
Mississippi	77,400	242,446	165,046	213.2%	18,147	92,136	72,910
North Carolina	248,235	881,068	632,833	254.9%	-66,925	114,986	517,847
South Carolina	118,611	451,216	332,605	280.4%	-627	161,704	170,901
Tennessee	229,273	787,393	558,120	243.4%	-43,195	368,544	189,576
Texas	762,250	2,255,448	1,493,198	195.9%	648,009	368,302	1,124,896
Virginia	301,340	844,684	543,344	180.3%	-51,210	0	543,344
West Virginia	64,039	230,881	166,842	260.5%	61,825	79,473	87,369
Connecticut	747,912	1,274,337	526,425	70.4%	0	0	526,425
Delaware	41,506	117,535	76,029	183.2%	273	0	76,029
District of Columbia	163,055	284,140	121,085	74.3%	0	0	121,085
Illinois	896,079	2,244,996	1,348,917	150.5%	0	634,080	714,837
Indiana	332,156	808,181	476,025	143.3%	22,473	71,194	404,831
Maine	85,192	273,303	188,111	220.8%	-45,218	45,135	142,976
Maryland	366,234	1,088,579	722,345	197.2%	0	84,500	637,845
Massachusetts	868,024	2,031,237	1,163,213	134.0%	0	239,976	923,237
Michigan	798,777	1,759,373	960,596	120.3%	-52,278	233,544	727,052
Minesota	502,161	936,086	433,925	86.4%	19,889	19,276	414,649
New Hampshire	67,270	552,594	485,324	721.5%	-53,923	371,525	113,799
New Jersey	664,632	2,623,009	1,958,377	294.7%	0	0	1,958,377
New York	4,285,230	10,167,635	5,882,405	137.3%	0	290,400	5,592,005
Ohio	861,365	2,151,074	1,289,709	149.7%	124,170	365,674	924,035
Pennsylvania	972,153	2,666,880	1,694,727	174.3%	7,197	500,140	1,194,587
Rhode Island	122,083	339,424	217,341	178.0%	-21,676	16,350	200,991
Vermont	33,805	97,021	63,216	187.0%	-13,404	9,431	53,785
Wisconsin	451,640	810,879	359,239	79.5%	56,229	25,015	334,224
Alaska	41,467	96,245	54,778	132.1%	0	0	54,778
Arizona	41,764	511,711	469,947	1125.2%	4,239	0	469,947
California	2,497,391	6,497,094	3,999,703	160.2%	0	1,188,250	2,811,453
Colorado	164,109	432,891	268,782	163.8%	44,711	151,657	117,125
Hawaii	71,733	149,709	77,976	108.7%	4,749	17,148	60,828
Idaho	26,702	78,378	51,676	193.5%	10,259	0	51,676
Iowa	160,263	334,801	174,538	108.9%	56,444	0	174,538
Kansas	141,244	418,847	277,603	196.5%	91,255	2,194	275,409
Missouri	234,747	729,330	494,583	210.7%	4,000	194,843	299,740
Montana	40,811	83,126	42,315	103.7%	14,858	1,255	41,060
Nebraska	85,691	170,734	85,043	99.2%	33,607	0	85,043
Nevada	42,104	203,329	161,225	382.9%	0	66,293	94,932
New Mexico	55,143	138,311	83,168	150.8%	27,677	8,163	75,005
North Dakota	56,564	67,632	11,068	19.6%	42,401	0	11,068
Oklahoma	220,793	338,097	117,304	53.1%	136,173	0	117,304
Oregon	117,470	324,577	207,107	176.3%	15,870	0	207,107
South Dakota	33,026	66,787	33,761	102.2%	11,535	0	33,761
Utah	56,175	107,987	51,812	92.2%	10,015	6,372	45,440
Washington	343,641	918,490	574,849	167.3%	96,585	66,104	508,745
Wyoming	17,029	39,592	22,563	132.5%	23,435	0	22,563
South	3,275,879	10,556,081	7,280,202	222.2%	818,114	2,266,771	5,013,431
Northeast	12,259,274	30,226,283	17,967,009	146.6%	43,732	2,906,241	15,060,768
West	4,447,867	11,707,668	7,259,801	163.2%	627,814	1,702,278	5,557,523
U.S.	$19,983,020	$52,490,032	$32,507,012	162.7%	$1,489,661	$6,875,291	$25,631,721

Note: "Devices" refers to provider specific taxes, voluntary contributions, and intergovernmental transfers, reported to HCFA in February 1992. It is assumed that most of the other sources for the state match are broad-based taxes.

survive the recession without a serious tax increase. At the other extreme, states such as Virginia received nothing.

The federal government has placed limits on the ability of states to generate Medicaid grants in this fashion and further limits on states' abilities to allocate these funds through the disproportionate share mechanism. These limits, enacted in the Medicaid Voluntary Contribution and Provider Specific Tax Amendments of 1991, are currently being implemented, and a great deal of uncertainty exists. The limits on financing mechanisms primarily restrain the growth in such vehicles in the short term. It is too early to predict the outcome of changes in the years ahead.

The greatest uncertainty surrounds the 12 percent ceiling placed on payments to providers servicing disproportionate shares of Medicaid and other poor patients. The state-by-state hold-harmless provisions built into the legislation almost certainly will total more than 12 percent, and it is unclear which ceiling(s) the Administration will elect to choose as controlling.

CONCLUDING OBSERVATIONS

This country's system of fiscal federalism is undergoing massive change. The growing dominance of Medicaid and other payments for individuals is dramatically changing the distribution of grant-in-aid funds. It is moving the locus of decisionmaking on appropriations away from Congress and state legislatures to unelected officials in the executive branches of government. While the experience varies substantially in different states, the change is increasingly blurring the checks and balances of our federal system.

Most states entered the 1990s with substantial recession-induced budget problems. They were faced with a federal government looking inward at its own problems that was unconcerned about states' problems in providing services to the public. To the contrary, Washington seemed intent on annually imposing new requirements on state and local governments, reducing state flexibility, *and* off-loading what had been federal costs. A federal government that saw itself without resources continually found ways to direct state government resources.

State political actors raised taxes and reduced and deferred spending. In half these states, they also looked to the one source of potential federal aid increase—Medicaid. The states created financing structures that permitted them to improve health services or increase payments to providers at small cost to the states themselves. Health services previously financed entirely with state or local government funds now received a federal Medicaid subsidy. Some participating states used financing vehicles primarily to expand their health care programs to underserved populations or communities. Others used them to better distribute the costs of health care to the poor over the entire health care community. Some states clearly saw these mechanisms as a means of generating additional federal dollars for their budgets, albeit partially to pay for new mandates. Some ignored or were ignorant of the mechanisms. Most states had mixed objectives.

Medicaid increases over the past half-decade have created fiscal problems for most states. In other states, the availability of new financing mechanisms has permitted expansion without significant cost. The Omnibus Budget Reconciliation Act of 1990 (OBRA 1990) purportedly resolved this issue when it definitively approved the use of provider-specific taxes but set limits to the use of voluntary contributions. When the Administration threatened that apparent certainty with aggressive regulations, the Medicaid Voluntary Contribution and Provider Specific Tax Amendments of 1991 placed ceilings on the use of financing vehicles. However, this solution may not be any more definitive than the "final" resolution enacted in 1990, and its main function may be to create avenues for assisting states in a recession without new spending legislation. The Medicaid program, with its entitlement status and open-ended "indefinite" appropriation, provided a vehicle for helping state political actors without specific congressional approval.

The recovery from the 1991 recession will not create substantial fiscal opportunities for most states. The federal share of Medicaid and AFDC costs will shrink automatically as the matching rates decline. Increases in own-source state revenues will be needed to liquidate the substantial inventory of unpaid bills, to provide deferred increases in employee compensation and welfare benefits, and to reinstitute programs of maintenance, etc.

The continued failure of the federal government to reduce deficit spending has produced a wide consensus to cap or reduce the unlimited access of entitlement programs to the federal treasury. A constitutional amendment that failed this year will be among the first agenda items of the new Congress. Alternative budget reforms will also be introduced, and final action is expected early in the session. All major budget proposals to date would for the first time either cap Medicaid or expose it to a sequester (14).

Without a health reform proposal that limits increases in federal health costs, an overall budget reform may well perform that function. A Medicaid sequester could unreasonably expose the states to unexpected cost shifts in the middle of a fiscal year. A simple ceiling could expose beneficiaries to a sudden loss of important benefits, or bankrupt certain classes of providers. It is clear that a health reform process is the more desirable mechanism. Whichever vehicle finally limits the drain of health costs on the federal Treasury, it would be hoped that these limits would be imposed in a manner least harmful to those that Medicaid is designed to serve, and least harmful to the federal system that has served this country well.

REFERENCES AND NOTES

1. Office of Management and Budget, Circular A-11 (Washington, D.C.: U.S. Government Printing Office).
2. Much of the section is derived from various publications of the U.S. Advisory Commission on Intergovernmental Relations (ACIR).

3. Advisory Commission on Intergovernmental Relations, Fiscal Balance in the American Federal System (Washington, D.C.: ACIR, 1967).

4. The relative decline in 1974–1975 reflects more the acceleration of other federal spending than a decline in grants.

5. However, the perceived need to limit highway spending outside the im poundment control process led to the imposition of today's highway obligation ceiling.

6. The increase to 17 percent in 1973 represents a group of one-time factors, including a double payment of initial general revenue sharing funds and acceleration of AFDC payments for 1974.

7. Budget authority is the authority, usually in the form of an appropriation, to commit the federal government to spend money.

8. This chapter makes some marginal changes in the federal budget concept treatment of payments for individuals. In particular, it excludes health block grants and includes aid to reimburse states for the health, welfare, and education costs of legalizing aliens (state legalization impact assistance grants).

9. This was the latest year available at the time this chapter was written. It precedes the extraordinary growth Medicaid has begun to experience in the 1990s.

10. These were the latest data available.

11. The following sections on state fiscal posture and response and Tables 10–14 are derived from Miller, V.J., Medicaid Financing Mechanisms and Federal Limits: a State Perspective (Prepared for the Robert Wood Johnson Foundation), July 1992.

12. National Association of State Budget Officers, Fiscal Survey of the States, April 1992. Financial analysts look for a 5 percent balance as an indicator of fiscal health.

13. The 1994 FMAPs are projected on the basis of preliminary per capita income data and should be used with caution.

14. A sequester is an automatic across-the-board reduction in budgetary resources to reach certain statutory goals. At present, Medicaid spending is totally exempt from sequesters.

•

6

The State Budget Context:
How Medicaid Fits In

STEVEN D. GOLD

Medicaid has been called the "Pac Man"® of state budgets, eating up ever larger shares of available resources and causing extreme fiscal stress and tax increases. Is this assertion true, or is it an exaggeration?

In order to provide a basis for answering this question, this chapter examines Medicaid's place in state budgets, reviewing its growth in relation to that of other major programs. It also analyzes changes in state tax systems and other revenues to determine whether states have been imposing greater burdens on their citizens in response to the fiscal pressures on their budgets. Although the chapter focuses primarily on past trends, it also addresses the likely consequences for other programs and the tax burdens of continued rapid escalation of Medicaid costs.

A major theme of this chapter is that many states have structural deficits, with the spending necessary to maintain current services and comply with federal mandates tending to fall persistently short of revenue from their existing tax systems. The growth of Medicaid spending is not the only source of state fiscal stress, but it is perhaps the largest single cause of these prospective deficits.

OVERVIEW OF STATE BUDGETING

There are countless ways to describe state budgets. By the broadest measure, in 1990 the U.S. Census Bureau reports that the states spent $572 billion and had revenues of $625 billion. The National Association of State Budget Officers (NASBO) reported total spending that year of $501 billion. The most commonly cited measure of state spending is for the general fund, which was $267 billion according to NASBO and $284 billion according to the National Conference of State Legislatures (NCSL) (1).

The amount of total state spending is not just a curiosity. If we want to know what proportion of state spending Medicaid represents, we must have a figure for total spending.

How do we get from $572 billion to $267 billion—more than a 50 percent reduction? The Census Bureau makes a distinction between general spending ($508 billion) and all other spending ($64 billion). More than 80 percent of the non-general spending is insurance trust expenditures—primarily pension payments to retirees but also unemployment benefits, workers compensation, and so forth.

The difference between the Census Bureau's measure of general spending and what states refer to as their general fund arises from several sources. The general fund does not generally include:

- Spending financed by federal aid ($126 billion in 1990).

- Spending paid for by user charges such as college tuition and highway tolls ($43 billion).

- Spending paid for by earmarked taxes.

What the general fund does include is most of the spending that is financed by taxes. But there is no standard definition of the general fund; each state defines it in its own way. In most cases, there is a myriad of other funds for specialized purposes as well.

NASBO reported that the states spent $62.4 billion on Medicaid in 1990. Approximately 57 percent ($35.8 billion) was federal aid. Of the state share ($26.5 billion), about 96 percent came from the general fund. [These figures do not include administrative costs, and they also exclude local Medicaid expenditures. (2)]

This discussion implies that there are several ways to measure the share of state spending devoted to Medicaid. Three of the leading possibilities are:

- Total Medicaid spending as a proportion of total state spending (as defined by NASBO).

- Medicaid spending excluding federal aid as a proportion of total state spending excluding federal aid.

- Medicaid spending from the general fund as a proportion of total general fund spending.

If one is concerned with the burden of Medicaid on state budgets, it makes sense to focus on the third measure, which excludes federal aid and spending in earmarked programs that are not supported by taxes. Nevertheless, the figure emphasized by NASBO and the National Governors' Association is the first measure, which includes federal aid.

Table 1 shows several different measures of the share of state spending devoted to Medicaid. In all cases, the share has been rising steadily. These figures may not convey the true role of Medicaid in recent state fiscal crises because for that purpose it is necessary to focus on the margin: Increases in Medicaid are consuming a larger share of the increment of tax revenue available to states for all programs. For example, NCSL estimated that

Medicaid appropriations for fiscal year 1992 were $6.4 billion higher than spending in the previous year. This represented 46 percent of the total increase in appropriations compared to 1991 spending (3).

Table 1. Alternative measures of the share of Medicaid in state budgets.

NASBO data			
Year	Percentage of all Spending	Percentage of all Spending Excl. Federal Aid	Percentage of General Fund Spending
1991 est.	13.6%	7.5%	10.5%
1990	12.5	6.8	9.5
1989	11.3	6.3	9.0
1988	10.8	5.6	8.7
1987	10.2	5.4	8.1

NCSL data	
	Percentage of General Fund
1992	12.0%
1991	10.4
1990	9.5
1989	9.0

Sources: National Association of State Budget Officers, *State Expenditure Report* (Washington, D.C.: various years); Eckl, C.L., Hutchinson, A.M., and Snell, R.K. *State Budget and Tax Actions 1991* (Denver, CO: National Conference of State Legislatures, 1991), and earlier editions of this report with various authors.

Note: There are some important differences between NASBO and NCSL data. NCSL figures for 1992 are appropriations in the budget enacted before the start of each fiscal year. Because many states enact supplemental appropriations for Medicaid, this is likely to understate the share of Medicaid spending in total budgets. In addition, in several states NCSL includes school aid in its figures for general fund spending even though aid is financed by an earmarked school fund. By contrast, NASBO figures are actual spending reported after the completion of the fiscal year, except in 1991, for which NASBO figures are estimates.

STATE EXPENDITURES

Table 2 shows the seven major categories of state expenditures and how they have fared since 1976. In order to remove the effects of inflation and show how spending fluctuated relative to the growth of the economy, spending has been expressed as dollars per $100 of personal income. To reveal how states have spent tax dollars, spending financed by federal aid and user charges has been subtracted (4).

Table 2. State spending per $100 of personal income excluding spending paid for by federal aid and user charges, 1976 to 1992.

Year	Total	Higher Education	Elem-Sec Education	Medicaid	Other Welfare	Health & Hospitals	Highways	Corrections	Other
1992p	$7.95	$0.84	$2.38	$0.79					
1991	7.80	0.86	2.34	0.66					
1990	7.91	0.90	2.31	0.61	$0.39	$0.64	$0.64	$0.40	$2.04
1989	7.86	0.90	2.32	0.60	0.40	0.63	0.64	0.37	1.94
1988	7.67	0.91	2.32	0.56	0.37	0.62	0.66	0.35	2.08
1987	7.55	0.92	2.33	0.55	0.39	0.61	0.66	0.33	2.06
1986	7.37	0.93	2.30	0.55	0.38	0.61	0.63	0.33	1.94
1985	7.28	0.92	2.23	0.56	0.38	0.59	0.60	0.30	1.98
1984		0.90	2.18	0.56	0.41	0.57	0.59	0.27	1.87
1983		0.90	2.17	0.51	0.36	0.59	0.60	0.25	1.83
1982		0.91	2.18	0.49	0.44	0.60	0.61	0.24	1.79
1981	7.43	0.93	2.29	0.45	0.51	0.62	0.65	0.23	1.71
1980	7.41	0.94	2.37	0.41	0.51	0.60	0.74	0.22	1.57
1979	7.28	0.94	2.31	0.38	0.51	0.58	0.72	0.21	1.60
1978	7.27	0.97	2.28	0.38	0.61	0.59	0.70	0.21	1.53
1977	7.49	0.96	2.29		0.60	0.61	0.69	0.20	1.76
1976	7.68	0.97	2.35	0.33	0.68	0.60	0.83	0.19	1.72

Source: Unless otherwise noted, U.S. Census Bureau, State Government Finances in (year) (Washington, D.C.: U.S. Government Printing Office, various years); for higher education, Center for Higher Education, Illinois State University, Grapevine; for elementary-secondary education, National Education Association, Estimates of School Statistics (annual) (Washington, D.C. various years); for Medicaid, U.S. Health Care Financing Administration.

Note: These figures are preliminary and are likely to be revised somewhat.

In a nutshell, the two growth areas of state spending have been Medicaid and corrections, both of which at least doubled relative to personal income between 1976 and 1990. Over the entire 14-year period, the lagging areas have been non-Medicaid welfare spending, highways, and higher education. The major reductions in those three areas occurred between 1976 and 1983. From 1983 to 1990, spending for these programs generally maintained its level relative to the overall economy.

Elementary-secondary education

School aid is by far the largest component of state budgets. It was depressed in the early 1980s as states suffered from fiscal stress, but it rebounded after 1983 as concern about school quality grew following publication of the report *A Nation at Risk.* Enrollment changes are an important influence on school spending. Enrollment fell 14 percent from 1973 to 1984, reflecting the baby bust that followed the baby boom. As children of the baby boom generation produce their own children, enrollment has begun to rise again. The National Center for Education Statistics (NCES) estimates that public school enrollment will grow 13 percent in the 1990s (5). This is an important change from the early 1980s, the last time the nation experienced a recession. At that time, enrollments were falling about one percent per year. Now they are growing by at least that much, adding to state fiscal stress. As Table 2 shows, state spending on elementary and secondary schools rose slightly faster than personal income in 1991 and 1992. This at first appears to be a surprisingly strong performance in view of the publicity about cutbacks during the recession. It reflects not only higher enrollments but also that schools are a high priority for states. To place this performance in perspective, it is helpful to consider the actual numbers underlying the figures in Table 2. In fiscal 1992, state spending for schools is estimated to have risen 4.8 percent while personal income was up 3.2 percent. Considering that enrollment was up 1.5 percent and inflation was about 3 percent, real spending per student was virtually unchanged. Thus, the increase in Table 2 is somewhat misleading: schools suffered, like most other programs, as a result of fiscal stress and demographic changes (6).

Higher education

In the early 1980s, an important shift began in state support of colleges and universities, requiring students to pick up a bigger share of the cost of their education. In the previous decade, state appropriations for higher education usually rose faster than tuition, but since 1982 the opposite has been the pattern (7).

This trend accelerated in the early 1990s. In the 1991–92 school year, state appropriations of tax dollars actually fell for the first time in more than 30 years, and average tuition rose more than 12 percent (8).

Non-Medicaid welfare programs

Welfare programs include both income maintenance (Aid to Families with Dependent Children, general assistance, and Supplemental Security Income) and services for the poor. Both categories fared very badly from

1976 to 1983, and income maintenance has continued to grow slower than personal income as benefits lagged behind inflation, but overall these programs have apparently kept up with personal income growth since 1983.

Health and hospitals

Spending on health and hospitals (other than through Medicaid) has grown slightly faster than personal income, reflecting two offsetting trends. Hospital spending rose relatively slowly, reflecting deinstitutionalization and privatization, but health spending more than compensated (9).

Highways

Spending for roads and streets rebounded in the mid-1980s following a sharp decline, but it did not attain the level relative to personal income that it had reached in the late 1970s. Highway spending differs from the other programs discussed here because it usually is funded by earmarked taxes. Therefore, it is not in direct competition for funds with Medicaid as other programs are.

Corrections

States went on a prison-building binge in the 1980s as they implemented tougher sentencing laws, prescribing mandatory prison terms for crimes that formerly often did not result in imprisonment. As a result, corrections spending was the fastest growing part of state budgets in the 1980s. Although its growth has been surpassed by Medicaid in the 1990s, corrections spending continues to rise significantly.

Trends since 1990

The national recession began in July 1990, the first month of fiscal year 1991 for most states (10). Since then the growth of Medicaid accelerated at the same time that revenue growth was slowing. Although spending trends in fiscal years 1991 and 1992 are not as well documented as those for earlier years, it appears that all categories of the budget were adversely affected by the fiscal stress that afflicted most states:

- Higher education was the biggest loser, suffering a small absolute decrease in state funding in fiscal year 1992.

- Elementary-secondary education continued to rise, but the increase in real per student spending fell close to zero, the smallest increase in state funding since 1983.

- Corrections spending continued to grow, but at a somewhat diminished rate. It increased at less than a double-digit rate for the first time since at least the early 1980s.

- Welfare benefits were cut in many states, either by reducing eligibility for general assistance or making absolute cuts in benefits. Only a small number of states raised benefits to reflect inflation. On the other hand, welfare rolls grew more than 20 percent as the recession boosted the poverty rate (11).

- Many state employees went without raises. In fiscal year 1992, 23 states did not provide across-the-board increases to reflect increases in the cost of living.

It is widely believed that the growth of Medicaid spending has to some extent come at the expense of other programs. As the discussion above shows, it is not common for spending for other programs to be cut in absolute terms. Rather, Medicaid has reduced funding increases for those other programs.

Three important qualifications are needed:

- This analysis has focused on national trends. Cutbacks occurring in some states have been obscured by increases elsewhere.

- The adverse impact of Medicaid on other programs has been particularly severe since 1990, but national data are incomplete for this recent period.

- One area where the growth of Medicaid appears directly related to shrinking support is income maintenance. Although welfare benefits were rarely cut in nominal dollars until 1991, they were sharply reduced in real dollars in the 1970s and 1980s.

STATE REVENUES

States obtain most of the revenue to fund services from three sources: taxes, charges, and federal aid. Taxes account for nearly two thirds of the total, charges for close to one tenth, and federal aid for about a quarter. Although the composition of state revenue changed somewhat in the 1980s, the level of revenue relative to the size of the economy in 1990 was about the same as it had been in 1980. As Table 3 shows, the sum of revenue from taxes, charges, and federal aid was $10.58 per $100 of personal income in 1990, only a little less than $10.66 in 1980. The most important changes in the composition of revenue were:

- A decrease in federal aid from $3.06 to $2.71 per $100 of personal income.

- A rise in charges from $0.82 to $0.98 per $100 of personal income.

- A small increase in tax revenue from $6.78 to $6.89 per $100 of personal income.

Table 3. State general revenue from taxes, charges, and federal aid, per $100 of personal income, 1980 and 1990.

Revenue	1980	1990
Total	$10.66	$10.58
Federal aid	3.06	2.71
Taxes	6.78	6.89
Charges	0.82	0.98
Exhibit:		
taxes+charges	$7.60	$7.87

Sources: U.S. Census Bureau, *State Government Finances*, (Washington, D.C.: U.S. Government Printing Office, various years); U.S. Department of Commerce, *Survey of Current Business* (various issues).

The changes in the composition of tax revenue were somewhat more dramatic, as Table 4 shows. Between 1980 and 1990, the personal income tax jumped from $1.84 to $2.21, and the general sales tax increased from $2.14 to $2.29. The growth in these taxes was offset by weakness in the corporation income tax (which fell from $0.67 to $0.50) (12) and severance taxes, primarily on oil production (down from $0.21 to $0.11). In other words, taxes shifted away from those that initially impact businesses to those that hit households directly.

Underlying these statistics are several important developments:

■ The relatively modest decrease in federal aid resulted from three offsetting trends: (1) Many programs providing aid directly to states were cut or grew at less than the inflation rate; but (2) the Medicaid program expanded so rapidly that it offset much of the decline in other aid programs; and (3) some aid programs were changed from federal-local to federal-state programs, with states distributing the funds to localities. Federal aid to local governments fell much more sharply than to states (13).

■ The general sales tax—still the largest single producer of tax revenue for most states—did not perform very well. If it were not for tax rate increases, sales tax revenue would have lagged behind the growth of personal income. The growth of the service sector—much of which is exempt from the sales tax— is the single biggest culprit underlying sluggish sales tax growth.

■ Corporation income tax revenue grew much more slowly than other major taxes, even if the cyclical drop in 1990 is disregarded. Among the reasons are the slow growth of profits and more aggressive efforts by corporations to minimize their tax liability. Although the average corporate tax rate increased

Table 4. State and local tax revenue per $100 of personal income, 1970 to 1992.

Fiscal Year	Total	Local	State	General Sales	Personal Income	Corporation Income	Severance	Other
							State	
1992	$11.15	$4.52	$6.90	$2.31	$2.20	$0.45		
1991	11.47	4.59	6.65	2.22	2.12	0.45		
1990	11.55	4.55	6.90	2.29	2.21	0.50	$0.11	$1.79
1989	11.60	4.57	7.02	2.31	2.20	0.59	0.10	1.83
1988	11.48	4.48	7.05	2.32	2.13	0.58	0.12	1.88
1987	11.24	4.37	7.02	2.26	2.16	0.59	0.12	1.89
1986	11.28	4.34	6.89	2.26	2.04	0.55	0.19	1.85
1985	11.30	4.35	6.97	2.25	2.06	0.57	0.23	1.86
1984	11.31	4.35	6.96	2.21	2.09	0.55	0.26	1.85
1983	10.68	4.25	6.46	2.02	1.88	0.50	0.28	1.78
1982	10.59	4.12	6.49	2.01	1.82	0.56	0.31	1.79
1981	10.85	4.20	6.67	2.07	1.82	0.63	0.28	1.87
1980	11.02	4.26	6.78	2.14	1.84	0.66	0.21	1.93
1979	11.37	4.46	6.94	2.19	1.81	0.67	0.16	2.11
1978	12.08	5.01	7.10	2.21	1.82	0.67	0.16	2.23
1977	12.15	5.17	7.02	2.14	1.77	0.64	0.15	2.32
1976	11.98	5.17	6.85	2.10	1.65	0.56	0.16	2.38
1975	11.74	5.09	6.68	2.07	1.57	0.55	0.15	2.34
1974	11.93	5.16	6.81	2.07	1.57	0.55	0.11	2.51
1973	12.41	5.43	7.01	2.04	1.60	0.56	0.09	2.72
1972	12.24	5.51	6.77	1.99	1.47	0.50	0.09	2.72
1971	11.50	5.26	6.27	1.88	1.24	0.42	0.09	2.64
1970	11.32	5.07	6.29	1.86	1.20	0.49	0.09	2.65

Note: Revenue for each fiscal year is divided by personal income in the calendar year that ended during it. Figures for 1991 and 1992 are estimated by the Center for the Study of the States, relying on Census data for 1991 and its own surveys for 1992.

Sources: For tax revenue, U.S. Census Bureau, *State Government Finances* (Washington, D.C.: U.S. Government Printing Office, various years). For personal income, U.S. Department of Commerce, *Survey of Current Business* 67 (August 1987) p. 44; U.S. Department of Commerce, *Survey of Current Business* 68 (August 1988) p. 30.

somewhat, interstate competition to attract industry had a restraining effect on tax increases.

■ The strongest growth of the personal income tax occurred in the first part of the 1980s, as states boosted tax rates to fend off the threat of deficits. The federal income tax reform enacted in 1986 had a number of effects on state income taxes: (1) It raised revenue in some states because they conformed to the broader federal tax base, but many states avoided this windfall by cutting their own tax rates or boosting personal exemptions and standard deductions. (2) Because many states mimicked the federal reform by making their tax rate schedules flatter, the responsiveness of revenue to economic growth (what economists call the income elasticity of the tax) was reduced, meaning that states now receive less automatic revenue growth each year when output increases. (3) It made tax revenue more unstable because capital gains represented a larger share of the tax base.

■ The decrease in severance tax revenue caused by lower energy prices and decreased production was a particular problem for most of the eight states that relied heavily on such taxes.

As Table 4 shows, state tax revenue per $100 of personal income was on a plateau from 1984 to 1990, fluctuating within a narrow range. This constancy of the overall level of tax revenue must be considered in relation to two other developments:

■ Local taxes rose faster than personal income, increasing from $4.35 to $4.59 per $100 of personal income. This reflects the relatively slow growth of aid to local governments during the 1984–1990 period.

■ The growth of revenue reflects two phenomena—discretionary changes of tax rates and the automatic increases in revenue that occur in response to economic growth. On balance, states were raising tax rates. As Table 5 shows, there were modest net increases each year from 1985 to 1990. The failure of total revenue to grow faster than personal income suggests that, in the absence of tax increases, revenue would have grown slightly slower than the economy.

As Table 6 shows, state and local revenue from taxes and charges per $100 of personal income trended upward after 1982 until the economic weakness of 1990 and 1991 depressed it. Because of the large tax increases passed in 1990 and 1991, when the economy recovers, revenue will probably be higher relative to personal income than at any time in the 1980s. It is still somewhat less than the all-time peak reached in 1973 (coincident with the peak of public school enrollment), but the direction is higher. Before long, it will probably reach a record high.

Table 5. Net state tax changes by year of enactment, Fiscal Year 1964 to Fiscal Year 1990.

Calendar Year	Billions of Dollars	Percent of Annual Collections
1991	$14.4	4.8%
1990	9.2	3.2
1989	3.5	1.3
1988	0.6	0.2
1987	4.5	1.9
1986	1.1	0.5
1985	−1.3	−0.6
1984	2.3	1.2
1983	8.3	4.8
1982	2.9	1.8
1981	3.8	2.5
1980	0.4	0.3
1979	−2.0	−1.6
1978	−2.3	−2.0
1977	0.2	0.5
1976	1.0	0.9
1975	1.6	2.0
1974	0.4	0.5
1973	0.5	0.7
1972	0.9	1.5
1971	5.0	9.7
1970	0.8	1.7
1969	4.0	9.5
1968	1.3	3.6
1967	2.5	7.8
1966	0.5	1.7
1965	1.3	5.0
1964	0.1	0.5

Sources: For, 1991, Gold, S.D., "How Much Did State Taxes Really Go Up in 1991?", *State Tax Notes* (December 30, 1991), pp. 623–626. Eckl, C., et al., *State Budget and Tax Actions: 1990* (Denver, CO: National Conference of State Legislatures); The Tax Foundation, cited in Gold, S.D., "State Tax Increases of 1983: Prelude to Another Tax Revolt?", *National Tax Journal* (March 1984), p. 14.

Note: The second column shows tax increases legislated during a calendar year as a proportion of total tax revenue during the fiscal year that ends during that calendar year.

Table 6. State-local revenue from taxes and user charges per $100 of personal income, 1970 to 1989.

Year	State-Local			State			Local		
	Taxes	Charges	Total	Taxes	Charges	Total	Taxes	Charges	Total
1970	11.32%	1.94%	13.26%	6.29%	0.80%	7.08%	5.07%	1.14%	6.21%
1971	11.50%	2.05%	13.55%	6.27%	0.86%	7.13%	5.26%	1.19%	6.45%
1972	12.24%	2.11%	14.35%	6.77%	0.88%	7.66%	5.51%	1.23%	6.73%
1973	12.41%	2.14%	14.55%	7.01%	0.89%	7.89%	5.43%	1.26%	6.69%
1974	11.93%	2.12%	14.05%	6.81%	0.88%	7.69%	5.16%	1.24%	6.40%
1975	11.74%	2.12%	13.86%	6.68%	0.87%	7.55%	5.09%	1.26%	6.35%
1976	11.98%	2.24%	14.23%	6.85%	0.89%	7.75%	5.16%	1.35%	6.51%
1977	12.15%	2.19%	14.35%	7.02%	0.84%	7.85%	5.17%	1.36%	6.53%
1978	12.08%	2.16%	14.25%	7.10%	0.85%	7.94%	5.01%	1.32%	6.33%
1979	11.37%	2.18%	13.56%	6.94%	0.83%	7.77%	4.46%	1.36%	5.82%
1980	11.02%	2.19%	13.20%	6.78%	0.82%	7.60%	4.26%	1.37%	5.63%
1981	10.85%	2.23%	13.08%	6.67%	0.84%	7.50%	4.20%	1.40%	5.60%
1982	10.59%	2.23%	12.82%	6.49%	0.84%	7.33%	4.12%	1.39%	5.52%
1983	10.68%	2.35%	13.04%	6.46%	0.87%	7.33%	4.25%	1.48%	5.73%
1984	11.30%	2.44%	13.73%	6.97%	0.91%	7.88%	4.35%	1.53%	5.88%
1985	11.28%	2.40%	13.68%	6.99%	0.89%	7.87%	4.32%	1.52%	5.83%
1986	11.24%	2.42%	13.66%	6.91%	0.91%	7.82%	4.35%	1.52%	5.87%
1987	11.48%	2.44%	13.92%	7.04%	0.91%	7.95%	4.48%	1.54%	6.02%
1988	11.57%	2.51%	14.08%	7.04%	0.92%	7.95%	4.55%	1.60%	6.15%
1989	11.56%	2.58%	14.14%	7.03%	0.95%	7.98%	4.55%	1.63%	6.18%
1990	11.46%	2.64%	14.10%	6.89%	0.98%	7.87%	4.60%	1.66%	6.26%

Sources: U.S. Census Bureau, *Governmental Finances* (Washington, D.C.: U.S. Government Printing Office, various years);
U.S. Department of Commerce, *Survey of Current Business* (Washington, D.C.: U.S. Government Printing Office, various years).

Although official figures for revenues in fiscal years 1991 and 1992 are not yet available, the Center for the Study of the States has estimated tax revenues for this study. The sharp decrease in fiscal year 1991 helps to explain why states had such serious fiscal problems during that period. The rebound in fiscal year 1992 is attributable primarily to the tax increases passed in the previous year. Without those increases, revenue would have still been very depressed (14).

State officials sometimes argue that they have reached the limits of their ability to raise taxes. It is true that tax increases are often hard to sell to constituents, particularly when the average family's standard of living is stagnant or falling. After a large tax increase, a passage of at least several years is usually required before another increase is politically feasible. Moreover, competition among the states makes it more difficult to increase taxes. But there is no permanent objective ceiling on the level of taxation. Besides, if all states are subject to the same upward pressures on their spending, it will be easier to increase tax rates. That is what occurred in the 1960s, when state and local tax revenue per $100 of personal income rose more than 20 percent.

One caveat should be noted. Nearly half of the states have enacted a statutory or constitutional limitation on state spending or revenue. Although few of these limitations have been restrictive until now (the oldest one has been in effect only 15 years), they will become more of a problem for state budgeters in the 1990s if pressures to increase spending continue to grow. States may have to consider suspending or relaxing these limitations (15).

Enormous differences exist among the states in terms of their capacity to finance services and their fiscal effort in using available capacity. As Table 7 shows, Mississippi is in the worst position, with per capita fiscal capacity in 1988 equal to only 65 percent of the national average, according to the Representative Tax System (RTS) developed by the U.S. Advisory Commission on Intergovernmental Relations. At the other extreme, Alaska's capacity was 59 percent above average (16).

This goes a long way toward explaining why spending is so low in Mississippi, but it is not the whole story. Mississippi's fiscal effort in 1988 was also low, only 94 percent of the national average. Many other states with low capacity also have low effort, while some states with relatively high capacity have above-average effort. The figures in Table 7 are somewhat controversial, and the Representative Tax System can undoubtedly be refined, but these estimates are useful in demonstrating the large differences in capacity and effort among states (17).

Table 8, which shows state-local tax revenue per $100 of personal income in 1980 and 1990 in each state, demonstrates differences in tax effort using a different approach. In both years there was a great deal of dispersion in the level of tax revenue. States also differed considerably in the rate of change of tax revenue during the 1980s, with taxes rising faster than personal income in 42 states and more slowly in eight states.

Table 7. State fiscal capacity and effort in 1988, according to representative tax system.

(National Average = 100)

State	Capacity	Effort	State	Capacity	Effort
Alabama	76	84	Montana	85	102
Alaska	159	127	Nebraska	90	98
Arizona	99	96	Nevada	135	69
Arkansas	74	84	New Hampshire	126	66
California	116	94	New Jersey	124	101
Colorado	107	89	New Mexico	83	99
Connecticut	143	90	New York	109	152
Delaware	124	84	North Carolina	91	93
Florida	104	82	North Dakota	86	91
Georgia	94	89	Ohio	91	97
Hawaii	114	112	Oklahoma	89	89
Idaho	76	93	Oregon	91	99
Illinois	99	102	Pennsylvania	94	97
Indiana	87	93	Rhode Island	99	104
Iowa	83	113	South Carolina	79	96
Kansas	91	104	South Dakota	78	95
Kentucky	81	88	Tennessee	84	83
Louisiana	83	90	Texas	96	88
Maine	98	105	Utah	78	106
Maryland	109	108	Vermont	105	100
Massachusetts	129	94	Virginia	104	91
Michigan	95	112	Washington	98	102
Minnesota	104	112	West Virginia	78	88
Mississippi	65	94	Wisconsin	90	119
Missouri	90	86	Wyoming	123	94

Source: U.S. Advisory Commission on Intergovernmental Relations, *1988 State Fiscal Capacity and Effort* (Washington, D.C.: ACIR 1990).

OUTLOOK FOR THE 1990s

If the Medicaid program continues to operate as it has in recent years, it will place enormous stress on state finances. The Congressional Budget Office recently projected that state and local costs (excluding federal aid) would grow from $39.6 billion in 1991 to $95.1 billion in 1997. That estimate may be optimistic because it assumes that annual increases after 1993 will slow to about 12 percent per year.

The ability of states to absorb higher Medicaid costs in the 1990s depends on many factors. Four are particularly important—economic growth, federal policy, demographic changes, and their own policies (18).

Economic growth

If the economy grew robustly, that would do a great deal to relieve state fiscal stress. Most importantly, it would make revenue grow faster. It would also probably produce some net savings in spending, particularly because of lower welfare costs and a slower increase in Medicaid spending.

Table 8. State and local tax revenue per $100 of personal income, 1980 and 1990.

	Total			State			Local		
	1980	1990	Change	1980	1990	Change	1980	1990	Change
New England									
Connecticut	$10.01	$11.00	9.9%	$5.53	$6.59	19.1%	$4.47	$4.41	-1.4%
Maine	11.67	12.21	4.6	7.49	7.86	5.0	4.19	4.35	3.8
Massachusetts	13.14	10.82	-17.7	7.24	7.15	-1.3	5.91	3.68	-37.8
New Hampshire	8.57	8.37	-2.4	3.36	2.65	-21.1	5.21	5.71	9.7
Rhode Island	11.64	11.40	-2.0	6.82	6.88	0.9	4.82	4.52	-6.2
Vermont	11.68	12.21	4.5	6.76	7.17	6.0	4.92	5.03	2.4
Mid Atlantic									
Delaware	11.46	11.01	-3.9	9.38	9.08	-3.2	2.08	1.93	-7.2
Maryland	11.40	11.18	-1.9	6.76	6.54	-3.2	4.64	4.64	-0.1
New Jersey	11.06	10.62	-3.9	5.63	5.67	0.8	5.43	4.95	-8.8
New York	15.47	15.54	0.4	7.50	7.56	0.9	7.97	7.97	0.0
Pennsylvania	10.87	10.62	-2.3	6.78	6.36	-6.2	4.09	4.26	4.3
Great Lakes									
Illinois	10.74	10.95	2.0	6.14	5.87	-4.3	4.60	5.08	10.3
Indiana	8.58	10.25	19.4	5.66	6.91	22.1	2.92	3.33	14.4
Michigan	11.24	11.88	5.7	6.72	7.01	4.4	4.53	4.87	7.6
Ohio	9.04	11.01	21.8	4.93	6.40	30.0	4.12	4.61	12.0
Wisconsin	11.80	12.77	8.3	7.95	8.19	3.0	3.84	4.58	19.1
Plains									
Iowa	10.63	11.88	11.8	6.59	7.53	14.4	4.04	4.35	7.6
Kansas	10.04	11.04	10.0	5.82	6.44	10.6	4.21	4.60	9.3
Minnesota	12.31	13.11	6.5	8.60	8.87	3.2	3.71	4.24	14.2
Missouri	8.87	9.45	6.6	4.97	5.88	18.2	3.89	3.57	-8.2
Nebraska	10.92	11.43	4.7	5.90	6.08	3.1	5.02	5.35	6.6
North Dakota	10.12	11.20	10.6	6.81	7.56	11.1	3.32	3.64	9.7
South Dakota	9.79	10.29	5.1	4.87	5.11	5.0	4.93	5.18	5.2
Southeast									
Alabama	9.25	9.57	3.4	6.79	6.81	0.2	2.46	2.76	12.3
Arkansas	9.49	9.64	1.6	7.37	7.29	-1.1	2.12	2.36	11.2
Florida	8.94	10.10	13.0	5.82	5.94	2.1	3.12	4.16	33.3
Georgia	10.25	11.29	10.1	6.65	6.85	3.0	3.60	4.44	23.3
Kentucky	10.07	10.76	6.8	7.97	8.32	4.3	2.10	2.44	16.4
Louisiana	11.13	11.64	4.6	7.55	7.22	-4.4	3.58	4.42	23.5
Mississippi	10.09	10.58	4.9	7.79	7.80	0.1	2.30	2.78	21.0
North Carolina	10.38	11.12	7.1	7.60	7.88	3.7	2.79	3.24	16.4
South Carolina	10.39	11.38	9.5	7.89	8.22	4.2	2.50	3.16	26.5
Tennessee	8.99	9.40	4.5	5.63	5.85	3.8	3.36	3.55	5.7
Virginia	9.86	10.16	3.0	5.91	5.72	-3.3	3.95	4.44	12.5
West Virginia	11.08	12.22	10.3	8.71	9.73	11.7	2.37	2.49	5.1
Southwest									
Arizona	12.48	12.53	0.4	7.68	7.79	1.5	4.80	4.74	-1.3
New Mexico	11.96	12.75	6.6	9.69	10.03	3.5	2.27	2.72	19.8
Oklahoma	10.06	10.86	7.9	7.14	7.62	6.6	2.91	3.24	11.1
Texas	9.35	10.58	13.2	5.51	5.52	0.1	3.84	5.07	32.1
Rocky Mountain									
Colorado	10.62	10.89	2.6	5.54	5.27	-4.8	5.08	5.62	10.6
Idaho	9.77	11.31	15.8	6.73	8.19	21.8	3.04	3.12	2.5
Montana	12.24	12.64	3.3	6.78	7.56	11.5	5.46	5.08	-7.0
Utah	11.69	12.21	4.4	7.49	7.92	5.7	4.20	4.29	2.0
Wyoming	14.29	14.57	2.0	8.42	8.88	5.6	5.88	5.69	-3.2
Far West									
California	11.33	11.41	0.6	7.91	7.50	-5.3	3.42	3.91	14.2
Nevada	9.69	10.83	11.8	5.94	7.40	24.5	3.74	3.43	-8.4
Oregon	10.89	12.24	12.4	6.15	6.21	0.9	4.74	6.04	27.4
Washington	10.34	12.30	18.9	7.39	8.84	19.6	2.95	3.46	17.2
Alaska	33.37	19.62	-41.2	28.63	13.56	-52.7	4.74	6.06	27.9
Hawaii	13.65	14.00	2.6	11.06	11.37	2.8	2.60	2.63	1.5
National	11.00	11.46	4.9	6.76	6.87	2.2	4.24	4.65	10.5

Sources: U.S. Census Bureau, Governmental Finances (Washington, D.C.: U.S. Government Printing Office, various years); U.S. Department of Commerce, *Survey of Current Business*, various issues).

Unfortunately, economic growth is likely to be relatively slow. The labor force will grow slowly because of the small number of entrants resulting from the baby bust. Given the labor force growth, the expansion of the economy is limited by the increase in productivity, which has been relatively low since 1973. Unless it accelerates, economic growth will be relatively modest.

Federal policy

If the federal government adopts a constitutional amendment to balance the federal budget, this is likely to result in an increased number of mandates and a reduced level of federal aid to state and local governments. This would probably add significantly to state and local fiscal stress. In the absence of such an amendment, the prospect is for continuing imposition of new mandates and moderate reductions in real aid other than for Medicaid. Although it is difficult to measure the burden of mandates, it is estimated that those enacted in 1989–1990 will cost states about $3 billion per year (19).

Demographic change

Aside from the increased number of senior citizens over the age of 85 (which should add to Medicaid costs), the most important demographic development is the growth in the school-age population. As mentioned above, the NCES estimates that public school enrollment is projected to grow 13 percent in the 1990s.

State policies

States are not helpless to affect their own fiscal destiny. If they reform their tax and spending policies, they will be better able to cope with the fiscal pressures that they will confront.

The specific reforms that are needed vary from state to state depending on the shape of their existing policies. In tax policy, important reforms include broadening the tax base, making the tax system more balanced (that is, increasing reliance on underutilized tax bases), and increasing the responsiveness of tax revenue to economic growth. In policies affecting local governments, states should reconsider how functions are sorted out, revise aid programs, relax mandates, and provide more options for local governments to raise revenue themselves. In spending policy, states should act to enhance accountability, target resources better, and take better advantage of incentive mechanisms to improve resource usage (20).

If state and local governments were to raise taxes substantially, that would enable them to expand services, but their ability to enact tax increases is limited at a time when real household income is relatively stagnant (if not declining). Taxpayer resistance to tax increases is not as great when the average standard of living is growing steadily, as it did in the 1960s. Unfortunately, there is little reason to be confident that incomes will grow much more strongly than they did in the past decade.

In summary, continuation of current policies implies that fiscal stress is on the horizon for many states. If Medicaid costs grow 15 percent per year, corrections spending increases 10 percent annually, school enrollment rises at more than 1 percent annual rate, state employees receive compensation increases comparable to those in the private sector, and other services are maintained, total spending will grow faster than the economy. Yet, in many states, tax revenue tends to grow about in line with the economy, if not somewhat more slowly. The result is a persistent budget gap (21). Medicaid is clearly one of the primary causes of this dismal prospect.

In this fiscal environment, state and local taxes will probably rise faster than personal income. Even with tax increases, states will be hard-pressed to improve services. Programs with strong public support, such as programs to provide preventive health care for children and early childhood education, will probably continue to expand, but the ability of states to undertake costly new initiatives will be limited.

IMPACT OF MEDICAID ON TAXES AND OTHER PROGRAMS

There are no generally accepted estimates of how much Medicaid has resulted in higher taxes or lower spending for other programs. In his discussion of this issue, Harold Hovey has summarized the situation well:

> Determining the source of state money to finance Medicaid is not easy. Because (rightly or wrongly) the program is not perceived as having widespread support, legislators and governors never explicitly raise money for it. No legislature in history has cut education to fund Medicaid. No legislature has raised taxes to fund Medicaid. Legislators do raise money for education. They also call for sacrifices in other programs to "balance the budget" and seek tax increases for budget balance and to keep open the doors of State government. So the inquiry over where the Medicaid money comes from is inherently complex (22).

Hovey suggested that a reasonable way to estimate the impact of Medicaid on tax increases is according to Medicaid's share of total state spending increases, which he estimated to be about 20 percent in the late 1980s and on the order of 50 percent for tax increases enacted in 1991 (23).

He also suggested that Medicaid has probably had a greater impact in reducing spending on social services and welfare benefits than on the rest of the state budget, particularly when Medicaid is administered by the same agency that is responsible for those other social programs.

The impact of Medicaid on taxes and other programs is especially difficult to disentangle in the last two years for at least four reasons:

- Bootstrap financing—provider taxes and contributions along with the federal aid that they bring in—has made it possible to some extent to increase Medicaid spending without burdening the rest of the state budget. In fact, such creative financing schemes provided some states with revenue that they were able to use to avoid cutbacks in non-Medicaid programs. In calendar year 1991, federal aid to state and local governments jumped 15.5 percent, not because of new aid programs but to a considerable extent because of bootstrap financing (24).

- States have become more aggressive about shifting other health programs into the Medicaid program, where they are eligible for a higher federal matching rate. States have also expanded school health programs, relying on Medicaid to provide at least half of the funding.

- The recession had a severe impact on revenue in many states. Separating the impact of weak revenue growth from large Medicaid increases is very troublesome.

- Many states relied on fiscal gimmicks to help them comply with their balanced budget requirements. One such gimmick is to defer spending until the next fiscal year. Such shifts in outlays from one fiscal year to another distort spending in Medicaid, education, and other programs. Only by adjusting for such actions can one see the true fiscal choices that have been made by the states.

Despite these complexities, there is no doubt that Medicaid has been one of the most severe problems for state budgeters in the early 1990s. The prospect of continued strong Medicaid growth is one of the reasons why the fiscal situation of states is likely to remain stressful even after the economy has emerged from the recession.

CONCLUSION

The reliance on states to fund more than 40 percent of the Medicaid program, while allowing them considerable discretion about the scope of services and eligibility, has both positive and negative effects. On the plus side, it is widely appreciated that this arrangement fosters experimentation and innovation. But there are also several important fiscal implications that are problematic:

- The large differences in fiscal capacity among states imply that Medicaid will be far from uniform across the nation. Despite the fact that poorer states receive considerably greater federal aid per dollar of their own spending, high-capacity states tend to have more generous programs.

- Differences in fiscal effort may make differences in programming even wider.

- The ability of states to fund Medicaid depends not only on the relative size of their tax bases and their fiscal effort but also on their spending for other programs, such as schools and prisons. Efforts to improve the educational system and to "get tough on criminals" compete with funding for Medicaid.

- Conversely, the explosive growth of Medicaid limits the ability of states to undertake initiatives in other areas, such as expanding social services (for children, senior citizens, and persons with special needs), improving infrastructure, aiding local governments, and strenthening the system of higher education. Health programs for persons not eligible for Medicaid are among the casualties.

- The increasing cost of Medicaid tends to force up state and local taxes. Through mandates that require states to pay a substantial part of the price of Medicaid, the federal government avoids raising its own taxes but indirectly contributes to state and local tax increases.

Certainly there are major questions implicit in the heavy reliance on states to fund a significant part of Medicaid. One of the key issues facing the nation as it considers the future of Medicaid is how serious it considers these problems to be.

REFERENCES AND NOTES

1. U.S. Census Bureau, *State Government Finances in 1991* (Washington, D.C.: U.S. Government Printing Office, 1991); *State Expenditure Report: 1991* (Washington, D.C.: National Association of State Budget Officers, 1991); Eckl, C., Hutchinson, A., and Snell, R., *State Budget and Tax Actions 1991* (Denver, Co.: National Conference of State Legislatures, 1991).

2. Local governments contribute to Medicaid costs in 13 states. To discuss the burden of Medicaid spending on local budgets would require a major expansion of this study, taking into account the particular structure of local government in each state where Medicaid is partly funded by counties or cities. In 1990, states accounted for 98 percent of direct spending on vendor payments for medical care.

3. NCSL Medicaid figures are not supposed to reflect revenue from provider taxes or voluntary contributions. NCSL reported a Medicaid increase of 21.8 percent in fiscal year 1992, considerably less than the total increase estimated by the federal government, which is approximately 30 percent. Nevertheless, it should be emphasized that NCSL estimates in the past have differed considerably from actual spending increases because of the tendency in many states to underestimate the growth of Medicaid spending. The 46 percent figure is subject to considerable uncertainty because the data for certain states reported by NCSL reflect shifts of spending between fiscal years, distorting spending comparisons among years.

4. The table excludes spending not covered in the seven major categories because, as reported by the U.S. Census Bureau, much of it is for activities of authorities that operate with considerable autonomy; much of this spending is not debated annually as part of deliberations on the state general fund budget. The largest category of miscellaneous spending is interest payments. For example, authorities that help homebuyers by providing mortgages with low interest rates pay out a large amount of interest on their own bonded indebtedness.

5. Gerald, D.E., and Hussar, W.J., *Projections of Education Statistics to 2002* (Washington, D.C.: National Center for Education Statistics, 1991).

6. All figures on school spending are from National Education Association, *1991–92 Estimates of School Statistics* (Washington, D.C., 1992). These figures are preliminary and are likely to be revised somewhat.

7. Gold, S.D., "The Outlook for State Support of Higher Education," in Anderson, R., ed., *New Directions for Higher Education* (San Francisco: Jossey Bass, 1990), p. 6

8. *The Grapevine* (a monthly publication from the Center for Higher Education, Illinois State University); State of Washington, Higher Education Coordinating Board, *1991–92 Tuition and Fee Rates: A National Comparison* (1992).

9. Gold, S.D., "State Finances in the New Era of Fiscal Federalism," in Swartz, T.R., and Peck, J.E., ed., *The Changing Face of Fiscal Federalism* (Armonk, N.Y.: M.E. Sharpe), p. 111.

10. The only states with different months to begin their fiscal years are New York (April), Texas (September), Alabama (October), and Michigan (October).

11. U.S. Congress, House Committee on Ways and Means, *Overview of Entitlement Programs*, pp. 1202–1203. Another explanation for the decrease in real AFDC benefits is the growth of Food Stamp benefits. In 1991, more than a dozen states cut welfare eligibility or benefits levels, especially for general assistance. Shapiro, I., et al., *The States and the Poor: How Budget Decisions in 1991 Affected Low Income People* (Washington. D.C.: Center on Budget and Policy Priorities and Center for the Study of the States, 1991). See also Moffitt, R., "Has State Redistribution Policy Grown More Conservative?" *National Tax Journal* (June 1990), pp. 123–142, which argues that increases in Medicaid and Food Stamps are responsible for the real decrease in AFDC benefits.

12. Corporate revenue was depressed in 1990 by the economic weakness that preceded the recession, so in retrospect it may appear to have been abnormally low. Even before 1990, however, corporate revenue was a declining share of state tax collections.

13. Gold, S.D., "The Federal Role in State Fiscal Stress," *Publius*, Vol. 22(3) pp. 33–47.

14. State tax increases enacted in calendar year 1991 totaled about $14.4 billion. More than 30 states raised taxes to some extent, but most of those increases were relatively small. Only 12 states boosted revenue 5 percent. Two states—California and Pennsylvania—acounted for about two-thirds of the total $14.4 billion tax increase. Gold, S.D., "How Much Did State Taxes Really Go Up in 1991?" *State Tax Notes* (December 30, 1991), pp. 623–626. The Center for the Study of the States tracks fluctuations in revenue in its quarterly State Revenue Reports and separates increases due to legislative actions.

15. That has already occurred in California, where voters in 1990 approved a constitutional amendment to loosen its expenditure limit, which was more severe than those in most other states. Generally, the limitations restrict spending or revenue growth to the rate of increase of personal income.

16. Fiscal capacity is based on the revenue that would be generated if each state applied the average national tax rate to each of the major tax bases employed by state and local governments. U.S. Advisory Commission on Intergovernmental Relations, *1988 State Fiscal Capacity and Effort* (Washington, D.C.: ACIR, 1990).

17. The ACIR has itself devoted considerable effort to improving RTS. Its most recent effort attempted to incorporate differences in needs among states. Rafuse, R.W., *Representative Expenditures: Addressing the Neglected Dimension of Fiscal Capacity* (Washington, D.C.: ACIR, 1990).

18. This section summarizes Chapter 2 of *The State Fiscal Agenda for the 1990s* (Denver, Co.: National Conference of State Legislatures, 1990).

19. Fabricius, M., "More Dictates from the Feds," *State Legislatures* (February 1991), p. 28

20. Gold, S.D., *The State Fiscal Agenda for the 1990s* (Denver, CO: National Conference of State Legislatures, 1989); Gold, S.D., *Reforming State-Local Relations, A Practical Guide* (Denver, CO: National Conference of State Legislatures, 1989).

21. This conclusion is not universally accepted. In 1986, the U.S. Treasury Department projected large surpluses for state and local governments, but it failed to take account of growing Medicaid and corrections costs, did not allow for increases in real compensation for employees, and overestimated the responsiveness of tax revenue to the growth of the economy (referred to by economists as the income elasticity of the tax system). U.S. Department of the Treasury, *Federal-State-Local Fiscal Relations* (Washington, D.C.: U.S. Government Printing Office, 1986). Another skeptical view is provided in Hovey, H.A., "Who Pays When State Health Care Costs Rise?" in Advisory Committee on Social Security, *State Governments: The Effects of Health Care Program Expansion in a Period of Fiscal Stress* (Washington, D.C., 1991). A recent series of studies by Policy Economics Group of KPMG/Peat Marwick confirmed that the elasticity of numerous state tax systems is less than 1.0 or only slightly higher.

22. Hovey, "Who Pays When State Health Care Costs Rise?", p. 101.

23. Ibid., pp. 116, 120.

24. Sullivan, D.F., "State and Local Fiscal Position in 1991," *Survey of Current Business* 72 (March 1992), p. 37.

•

7

Medicaid Fiscal Stresses and the States: A Medicaid Director's Perspective

GARY J. CLARKE

INTRODUCTION

Almost from the inception of the Medicaid program in 1965 and through the mid-1980s, the standard fare for health policy analysts has been to blame most of the access problems of the United States on the shortcomings of the Medicaid program and its administration by the states. Medicaid agencies have often been characterized as beleaguered, belittled, and befuddled—the favorite whipping boys of policy analysts of all stripes. Whether it was low payment, lax utilization review, or inadequate eligibility standards, all the ills of the American health care system were laid at the feet of Medicaid agencies.

Remarkably, however, there has come a new awareness of both the importance of the Medicaid program in the American health picture and the difficulties of accomplishing national goals through this or any other program. Since the mid- to late-1980s, state Medicaid agencies have taken off in a burst of growth that has alarmed both state and federal analysts alike. Those federal analysts who called for expansion of services, increases in payment, and more generous eligibility are suddenly seeing the enormous costs associated with those changes. And despite the fact that Medicaid programs still have the lowest prices, the most efficient claims processing systems, the best fraud detection programs, and the most managed-care penetration of any large public health insurer in the country, the subject of "out of control" Medicaid growth is on the lips of every policy "wonk" within 100 miles of the Potomac River.

How did Medicaid suddenly grow from the most penurious to the fastest growing program in the state and federal governments? Was it policy mandates, or economic forces, or sudden generosity, or—as Bush Administration budget officials would have the public believe—state scheming? Has the expansion really helped anybody? Are the causes controllable? And are we headed down the wrong or right track? Indeed, is there any track or course at all? Navigating the Medicaid ship of state is like being tossed in an angry sea between the rocks of budget cutters on the right and reefs of patient and provider advocates on the left, with federal mines (regulations) all around. For the average Medicaid director, there is no course at all—only survival for a few years until the next seaman is hauled on deck for a turn at the wheel.

FIVE GENERAL TRENDS

From my perspective, five distinct policy trends have come together to thrust the Medicaid program into the forefront of government spending. The first (though scarcely now remembered) is the effort of the states themselves to break the welfare paradigm of Medicaid. When the Southern states became concerned about their infant mortality rates, they were the first important interest group to successfully lobby Congress to sever the paralyzing relationship between welfare eligibility and Medicaid. The permissive legislation of OBRA 1986 set off a tidal wave of mandates in 1987 and beyond. Thus, in a very real sense, the states asked for and received permission to engage in a good bit of the spending going on today.

The second, and by far the most important policy trend, is the succession of new legislation that started with OBRA 1987, and continued with the Medicare Catastrophic Coverage Act (May 1988), and then followed by OBRA 1988, 1989, and 1990. With these statutes, Congress turned options into mandates and invented far more requirements than states ever asked for. Good administrative inventions in one state—like "outposted" eligibility workers, or shortened application forms—suddenly became the mantra (and mandate) for reform in all states. Once the policy bubble of Medicaid was broken, the art of the possible suddenly became more wide open in Congress. Just as important, the cost of accomplishing national goals suddenly became a lot cheaper if states financed 45 percent of the cost (as they do, on average, in the Medicaid program). Moreover, many of the biggest states, such as California, Michigan, and New York, were easily kept at bay, since they already had more generous Medicaid programs and, for several years, were scarcely affected by mandates.

The third important trend affecting the growth of the Medicaid program has been the increasingly successful wave of legal services and provider litigation. The mandates of OBRA 1989 for instance, are a virtual paean to a law review article written by a legal services advocate advising how to secure additional rights under the Medicaid program. Recent federal court interpretations of the 1982 Boren Amendment (spurred by a variety of provider lawsuits throughout the country) have had the same effect. Decisions in various Boren cases have so tortured congressional history that collectively they probably signal a return to unlimited, cost-based institutional payment as just about the only reimbursement scheme certain to pass judicial muster.

The fourth important trend is increasing interest and concern about health care issues in state legislatures and governors' offices. This has been complimented by increasing professionalism and performance of state Medicaid agencies. States are no longer content to wait for federal leadership for health reform. If Medicaid is the only federal tool they have to expand health coverage, then it will be stretched to the maximum limits. No longer is it considered acceptable, or even possible, to have cost-shifting or state or local general revenues cover the costs of treating Medicaid patients. In addition, under the watchful but encouraging eye of their state legislatures, Medicaid administrators are working far more closely with their colleagues in other state and local agencies to match state funds with available federal Medicaid monies. So too, increasing emphasis on customer service is resulting in better and quicker payment in numerous states, encouraging, in turn, increased provider participation, better access, and increased expenditures.

The fifth and final trend, which may be even more important than federal mandates, is the deterioration of the economy, and in particular the inflationary health insurance economy—inflation from which the Medicaid program itself is not immune. This economic and private health insurance deterioration has made growth in the Medicaid program an almost impossible engine to stop. Far more people than ever imagined are in need of Medicaid's help. Either they do not have jobs, or the jobs they do have no longer come with any, adequate, or affordable health insurance. In Florida, for instance, the Hospital Cost Containment Board reported that in 1989, the decline in revenue from privately insured hospital patients—from 37 to 34 percent—was almost exactly made up for by the increase in revenue from Medicaid patients—from 6 to 9 percent.

In sum, then, we seem to have come to a point in history where policymakers, lawyers, agency administrators, and the economy have converged on the Medicaid program. The results, in terms of increased cost and coverage, are inevitable. "Out of control" are the words facile policy analysts use to describe the current data. But what they really mean is "growing faster than we wish"—for the results are surely what was intended. Far from being out of control, current growth in the Medicaid program is primarily a result of the policies we have chosen as a nation to adopt: whether it is the policy to increase eligibility; the policy to increase prices (particularly for most favored providers); the policy to *not* control overall health care inflation; the policy to *not* require health insurance as a condition of employment; or the policy to subsidize the shortcomings of Medicare through the Medicaid program. As the payor of last resort, Medicaid expenditures will inevitably rise as our other programs and policies fail. In essence, the proverbial "safety net" has been widened considerably in recent years to help both recipients and providers, and the "catch" is far bigger than ever imagined.

IMPACT ON A SOUTHERN STATE—THE FLORIDA CASE

The impact of these trends on the State of Florida's Medicaid agency has been tremendous. In the course of 12 state fiscal years, from 1980–81 to 1992–93, state and federal spending for the Medicaid program has risen almost tenfold—from $589 million to $5.4 billion (see Figure 1). This is an annualized average growth rate of 16 percent per year.

Using this same rate of growth in expenditures and projecting to the year 2000, total Medicaid spending is estimated to rise to $12 billion—more than doubling in a scant eight years. However, if the experience of only the last five years is trended forward, then the average annualized rate of growth is 29 percent per year. Using this figure, the effect of compounding results is a staggering estimate of $20 billion for the year 2000 (see Figure 2).

Changes in total Medicaid expenditures are mainly driven by four factors—changes in the total number of covered persons; changes in price or payment; changes in service coverage; and changes in patient utilization. At least in the Medicaid program, administrative costs are relatively insignificant. In Florida, it amounts to about five percent of the total, with more than 75 percent of that cost attributable to eligibility staff. Administrative costs for claims processing, policy development, utilization review, etc., are less than one percent and are declining on a per recipient or per claim basis.

Figure 1.

Florida Medicaid Program
Growth in Service Expenditures

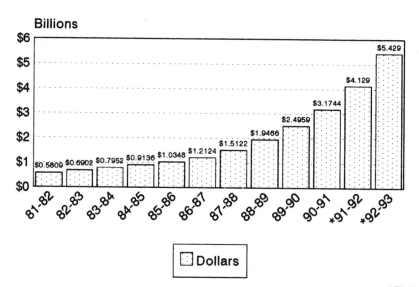

Billions

81-82	$0.5809
82-83	$0.6902
83-84	$0.7952
84-85	$0.9136
85-86	$1.0348
86-87	$1.2124
87-88	$1.5122
88-89	$1.9466
89-90	$2.4959
90-91	$3.1744
*91-92	$4.129
*92-93	$5.429

☐ **Dollars**

*Estimate

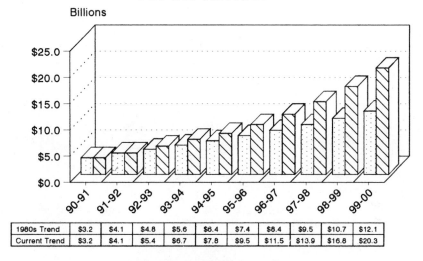

Projected Medicaid Budget For the Nineties

Billions

	90-91	91-92	92-93	93-94	94-95	95-96	96-97	97-98	98-99	99-00
1980s Trend	$3.2	$4.1	$4.8	$5.6	$6.4	$7.4	$8.4	$9.5	$10.7	$12.1
Current Trend	$3.2	$4.1	$5.4	$6.7	$7.8	$9.5	$11.5	$13.9	$16.8	$20.3

□ 1980s Trend ◩ Current Trend

Figure 2.

The following sections summarize the Florida experience in the four main areas of expenditure increase.

Changes in Eligible Population Groups

It is difficult for Florida to sort the effects of "federal mandates" from state interests. Florida was one of the first states to take advantage of the then optional opportunities of the Sixth Omnibus Budget Reconciliation Act (sometimes called SOBRA). In the first legislative session following SOBRA's enactment, the Florida legislature voluntarily extended coverage to pregnant women and children to age 2 to 100 percent of poverty (and waived assets tests); added elderly and disabled adults to 90 percent of poverty; initiated a presumptive eligibility program; and outstationed eligibility workers. In addition, it voluntarily reduced its application form to one page. All of these changes reflected increased commitment by the legislative and executive branches to increasing access to health care for poor Floridians. In addition, all of these early changes were financed by the hospital assessment first enacted in Florida in 1984.

In subsequent years, Florida voluntarily picked up elderly and disabled adults to 100 percent of poverty; children to their various maximums; and additional pregnant women—first to 150 percent and then 185 percent of poverty. It also complied with Qualified Medicare Beneficiary (QMB) mandates. These later changes were financed with a combination of "fund

Florida Medicaid Eligibles
Fiscal Year 1991-92

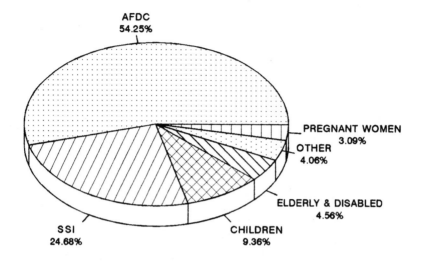

AFDC
54.25%

PREGNANT WOMEN
3.09%

OTHER
4.06%

ELDERLY & DISABLED
4.56%

SSI
24.68%

CHILDREN
9.36%

Figure 3.

shifts" from existing "general revenue only" programs, a nine-cent-per-pack increase in the state cigarette tax, and new general revenue increases.

The results of these eligibility changes are shown in Figure 3. Today, special categorical groups of Medicaid eligibles—virtually none of which existed in 1986—constitute 21 percent of the entire total. Children under ages 1, 6, and 9 (there are currently three different income eligibility levels), whose parents are not eligible for Medicaid assistance, comprise more than nine percent of the entire group. Elderly and disabled persons (92 percent of whom are also QMBs) are the next largest group at 4.6 percent, followed by pregnant women at 3 percent.

It is intriguing to note that in 1984–85, the year that Florida passed its hospital assessment, the total number of Medicaid recipients actually fell (see Figure 4). This was a result of a reduction in AFDC recipients, as well as the termination of a special Cuban refugee program. For the next two years, "other" groups were a virtually insignificant total, and Florida Medicaid was a barebones AFDC and SSI-only program as far as eligibility was concerned. July 1986 marked the beginning of a medically needy program for the first time in Florida. October 1987 marked the beginning of the first groups of SOBRA eligibles (pregnant women, children to age 2, and elderly and disabled).

Interestingly, as the groups of optional (now mostly mandatory) "other" groups grew, the number of medically needy fell. Today, after recent budget

Florida Medicaid Services
Growth in Eligibles

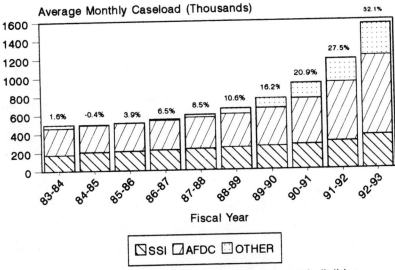

Percentages equal year to year changes in total eligibles

Figure 4.

cuts reducing the medically needy income level to the AFDC income standard (31 percent of poverty in Florida), the medically needy now comprise less than one percent of total recipients.

Perhaps the most interesting factor to note in Figure 4, however, is that the total number of Medicaid eligibles more than doubled in less than ten years, even without the new mandatory groups! This increase was mostly accounted for by an increase in AFDC recipients. In July 1985, the nadir of the program, the Florida AFDC Medicaid caseload stood at 291,205. By June 1992, that same caseload was estimated at 671,121—an increase of 230 percent in just seven fiscal years.

AFDC caseload growth in Florida is probably attributable to a number of causes. The most important recent cause is the significantly worsening economy. However, our anecdotal experience leads us to believe that an important factor was a new attitude about enrolling potential recipients, as well as modernized systems for doing so. For instance, the eligibility workers Florida outposted in hospitals, health departments, and community health centers reported finding just as many or more recipients fitting the AFDC category of eligibility as they did those fitting the "pregnant women," "children" or "medically needy" categories they were outstationed to find. In addition, a new management philosophy of customer service replaced a prior, mostly federally mandated concern with "error rates." This change in attitude is reported to have encouraged more persons to come through the door to submit an application.

Another anecdotally reported factor resulting in an increase in Medicaid recipients was the relative worsening of the health provider economy. As Medicare and other insurers began to tighten their reimbursement policies, health care providers of all stripes are reported to have gone to far greater lengths than previously to encourage their indigent and under-insured patients to apply for Medicaid assistance. This was especially true for hospitals, which beginning in 1984 in Florida contributed 1.5 percent of net revenues to expand Medicaid and other indigent health programs. In addition, in 1987, health departments, community health centers, and MCH administrators began placing a far greater premium on Medicaid eligibility, which has become their largest source of growth revenue.

Percentage Growth in Eligibles
Percentage Growth in General Revenue

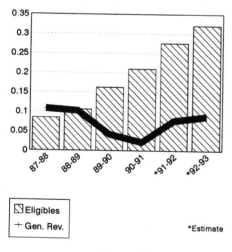

Eligibles
+ Gen. Rev.

*Estimate

Figure 5.

Figure 5 shows the startling effects of growth in Medicaid eligibles occurring simultaneously with the decline in state revenues caused by a worsening economy. As in any recession, state revenues decline as needs increase. In 1991, state revenues grew less than 4 percent, while Medicaid recipients increased by 21 percent. Had this occurred in 1987, the state could have reduced its optional groups as a way to balance its budget. By 1991 this policy flexibility was gone. (In Florida, less than one percent of all eligibles are now covered in an "optional" group.) Thus, state resources are diverted from other programs—primarily education and other human service areas—as a way to make ends meet.

Changes in Medicaid Prices

Despite their reputation as the lowest paying of all major insurers, state Medicaid programs are not immune from rampant health care inflation. In four out of the five largest categories of spending—hospitals, nursing homes, ICF/MRs, and ingredient costs of prescription drugs—prices are generally adjusted for inflation in all states. In Florida, these four categories

Projected Medicaid Expenditures
Fiscal Year 1991-92

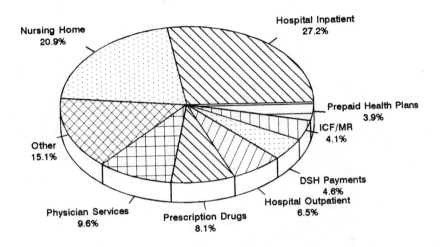

Figure 6.

account for 67 percent of all spending. In addition, HMO expenditures—driven largely by changes in hospital, physician, and drug prices and utilization—are also thus adjusted for inflation and account for another 5 percent. See Figure 6 for a breakdown of these expenditures.

Florida's institutional reimbursement methodologies during this period of time were not particularly strict compared to many states. Generally, they were (and are) cost-based prospective methodologies, with prospective payments tied to a regional or national inflation index published by Data Resources Inc. (DRI). In addition, retrospective adjustments are made to allow for additional expenses, subject to various limitations.

The remaining large category of expenditures is physician services at 9.6 percent. During the late 1980s, Florida made a major commitment to increase its physician prices to near Medicare parity (50th percentile) over a five-year period. With minor exceptions, however, all other prices were frozen during this time span.

As shown in Figure 7, overall price increases (inflation) in the Florida Medicaid program in the last five years have averaged right around 10 percent, with the exception of 1991–92 when new hospital controls and temporary nursing home controls were put into place. In addition, in late 1991 due to budget shortfalls, the legislature rolled back physician fee increases by 30 percent (with the exceptions of OB care and office visits).

Figure 7 shows the clear dilemma of Medicaid programs nationwide.

Percentage Growth in Price Level
Percentage Growth in General Revenue

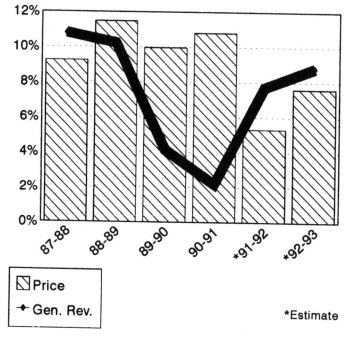

Figure 7.

When relatively generous (by Medicaid standards) reimbursement schemes are used, growth in health care prices exceeds growth in general revenue. This forces Medicaid programs to take a bigger and bigger portion of the state pie, even without any growth in eligibles.

States can (and have) take steps to limit growth in prices to levels below overall health care inflation. However, the threat or eventuality of "Boren amendment" litigation constrains these options. Indeed, this short statement of federal law has become, through court interpretation, tantamount to the latest in a long line of costly federal mandates. In essence, given new court holdings now being followed in multiple jurisdictions, the burden is now on the states to prove that anything but full cost reimbursement is acceptable. In addition, states must now comply with a host of new "due process"requirements never envisioned by Congress in its wildest imaginings, nor required by Health Care Financing Administration (HCFA) in its ten-year history of administering these provisions.

This same phenomenon of greater federal oversight is now being felt in the area of non-institutional physician provider reimbursement as well. OBRA 1989 requirements concerning adequate payment of obstetricians and pediatricians are literally worded to require states to pay "whatever it takes" to assure that private physicians work with Medicaid patients to the same degree they work with private patients. These requirements are imposed despite the development of MCH programs and community health centers, which frequently provide better care in a completely different manner; and despite the rapid development of Medicaid HMOs in many areas of the country that do not even receive fee-for-service reimbursement. Indeed, in some parts of Florida, the combination of county health departments, community health centers, and Medicaid HMOs has made private fee-for-service medicine largely irrelevant to the provision of care to Medicaid children and pregnant women.

To add insult to injury, in OBRA 1990 Congress actually explicitly forbade the reduction of prices paid to pharmacists for four years. This means that neither dispensing fees nor ingredient costs can be reduced during this period of time.

Thus, in the areas of Medicaid where states spend most of their money—institutions, prescription drugs, and (some) physician services—states are required to deal with an increasingly specific federal floor on prices. In Florida, these areas amount to about 83 percent of the total Medicaid budget.

Generally speaking, because these federal floors may be tied to health care inflation, they are higher than state revenue-raising capabilities. And unlike Medicare, the perversity of federal law subjects state Medicaid officials to potential personal liability (1983 civil rights actions) for reimbursing providers less than what they believe they are entitled to under these federal requirements. This liability exists despite the vagueness of the "Boren" standard, despite the fact these are more in the nature of societal judgments than personal civil rights, and despite the fact that these decisions are generally made in the legislative rather than executive arena. Only in the United States could a health care provider, who is free to enter or leave the Medicaid program at any time based on his own economic interests, sue a government official personally if he believed he was not being reimbursed adequately. Somehow, our notions of "free market enterprise" seem to go only one way when they apply to the Medicaid program. (See also, federal requirements on states as applied to "freedom of choice.")

Changes in Service

Recent state and federal changes in service definitions and requirements have also had a major impact on the growth of expenditures. While these changes are harder to clearly distinguish from changes in either price or utilization, they clearly are important factors.

One of the most important changes occurred in OBRA 1987, which established a clear requirement to define and make additional payments to "disproportionate share" hospitals. These additional payments in essence changed the definition of what was paid for during a Medicaid hospital stay—and made the state and especially federal cost for this program enormously larger. This same disproportionate share mandate unwittingly gave rise (for good and for bad) to state tax and donation schemes that spread like wildfire among the states from 1989 to 1991. (Under a "donation" program, a hospital "gives" the money to the state, which then uses it to draw down federal match. The state then returns to the hospital at least as much as money as it gave— without the hospital ever having served an additional patient!)

In some states, 25 percent of the entire Medicaid budget is devoted to disproportionate share payments—an amount only slightly less than the share devoted to all inpatient hospital Medicaid payments in Florida. Even with Florida's more conservative approach, almost $250 million in disproportionate share payments will be made in 1992–93, or about 4.7 percent of the total budget. Yet in state Fiscal Year 1987–88, such a fiscal category did not exist.

A similar service definition/payment requirement was created in OBRA 1989 with regard to federally qualified health centers (FQHCs). This program requires states to pay federally established community health centers on a cost basis for Medicaid recipients, resulting in most states in payments higher than fee-for-service rates for a similar service. While the incremental cost is relatively small, the precedent of paying most favored providers more than others was carried from the institutional (hospital disproportionate share) to non-institutional (FQHC) arena.

The most important change in federal Medicaid service requirements since the program was first enacted in 1965 occurred with the passage of OBRA 1989. One of the mandates of this new statute required that states pay for all medically necessary services defined in Section 1905(a) of the statute for children, regardless of whether these services are included in the state plan or not. Previously, most of the more penurious state Medicaid programs did not pay, or severely limited payment, for a variety of "optional" programs, such as physical and speech therapy, durable medical equipment, private duty nursing, and the like. In addition, many states, particularly in the South, had numerous arbitrary limits on such items as inpatient hospital care (typically, number of days per person per year) and outpatient hospital care (visits, or total expenditures per person per year). In one fell swoop, OBRA 1989 eliminated these cost-limiting portions of state Medicaid programs as they applied to children.

Figure 8 shows the estimated 1991–92 total impact of the new EPSDT service requirements for children mandated in Florida by OBRA 1989— $111.5 million. Moreover, when all other requirements of OBRA 1989 are considered, including expanded eligibility coverage, increased payments for obstetricians, increased hospice payments for patients in nursing homes, enhanced FQHC payments, and the cost of administration, the total 1991– 92 cost amounted to $204.3 million (Figure 9). In total, the state of Florida created nine new programs, amended seven others, and filed 33 separate state plan amendments in order to comply with OBRA 1989.

In many other states, the pharmacy "reforms" of OBRA 90, by requiring maintenance of an open formulary, significantly increased the services

Mandated EPSDT Expenditures (OBRA '89)

EARLY AND PERIODIC SCREENING,
DIAGNOSTIC AND TREATMENT
SERVICES DEFINED.

PERSONAL CARE	$ 746,504
SKILLED NURSING	860,725
DME	11,874,890
INPATIENT CAP ELIMINATION	46,174,357
OUTPATIENT CAP ELIMINATION	22,787,587
PHYSICAL THERAPY	1,616,505
OCC., SPEECH, RESPIRATORY THER.	2,887,184
TRANSPLANT COVERAGE	2,889,000
IMMUNIZATIONS	2,221,463
TPN	1,638,000
ANTI-HEMOPHILIAC FACTOR	678,150
PRIVATE DUTY NURSING	8,252,508
CASE MANAGEMENT (TARGETED)	8,890,477

TOTAL COST FOR EPSDT SERVICES	$111,517,350

Figure 8.

OBRA '89 — FY 1991–92 Total Expenditures

MANDATORY COVERAGE OF CERTAIN LOW INCOME PREGNANT WOMEN AND CHILDREN	$ 55,281,893
PAYMENT FOR OBSTETRICAL AND PEDIATRIC SERVICES	8,054,901
HOSPICE PAYMENT FOR ROOM AND BOARD	6,162,031
EARLY AND PERIODIC SCREENING DIAGNOSTIC AND TREATMENT SERVICES DEFINED	111,517,350
PAYMENT FOR FEDERALLY QUALIFIED HEALTH CENTER SERVICES	15,133,110
ADMINISTRATION	8,154,338

TOTAL COST	$204,303,623

Figure 9.

Medicaid Expenditures by Eligibility Group
Fiscal Year 1991-1992

ELIGIBILITY GROUP	AVG EXPEND MONTH/ELIG	ANNUAL EXPEND PER ELIGIBLE
Mandatory		
SSI (INSTITUTION)	$2,042.49	$24,507.48
SSI (OTHER)	$395.51	$4,746.12
AFDC	$128.02	$1,536.24
New to Florida since 1986		
MEDICALLY NEEDY	$605.64	$7,267.68
PREGNANT WOMEN	$440.37	$5,284.44
ELDERLY & DISABLED	$318.37	$3,820.44
CATEGORICALLY ELIGIBLE	$251.90	$3,022.80
CHILDREN	$221.11	$2,653.32

Figure 10.

provided in those states. These states also report that the increased costs of maintaining an open formulary were *not* offset by additional manufacturer rebates. Because Florida always maintained a primarily open formulary, except for certain high cost items, the state experienced a net fiscal gain. However, subsequent Florida attempts to gain further control of pharmacy expenditures have been opposed by litigation and lobbying efforts directed by out-of-state corporations, who rely on the mandates of OBRA 1990 to justify protection of their economic interests.

Changes in Utilization

The standard formula for determining total costs in the Medicaid program is average price per service, times total eligibles, times total services per eligible. The latter variable is more commonly recognized as utilization—a measurement of the number of times the average recipient uses a Medicaid service. (For ease of calculation to figure overall utilization, each service is given a value of 1—although some services are obviously more expensive than others.)

As a result of the eligibility changes made from 1986 through 1990, the Florida Medicaid program experienced an increase in services (and expenditures) per recipient. This was not surprising. By definition, medically

Percentage Growth in Utilization
Percentage Growth in General Revenue

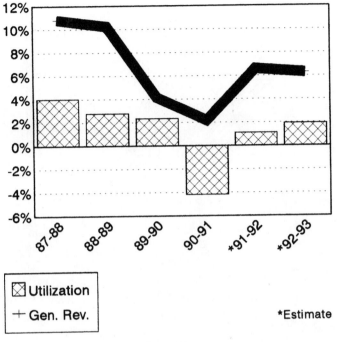

Figure 11.

needy recipients (added July, 1986) and pregnant women (added October 1987) used more services than the average Medicaid recipient. In fact, their average utilization even exceeded non-institutionalized SSI recipients. In addition, children under age one on Medicaid, who are disproportionately represented in hospital neonatal intensive nurseries throughout the state, also resulted in high use and expenditures. In fact, all the new groups had higher utilization and expenditures per recipient than the average AFDC recipient (see Figure 10).

Thus, the result of the eligibility expansions begun in 1986 not only increased total numbers of Medicaid recipients, they also changed the mix. By targeting those most in need of health care services (as the Southern governors had originally asked), states not only got more recipients, they got more costly ones. Far from being out of control, this was yet another deliberate policy decision intended to increase Medicaid payments—although reducing infant mortality was our ultimate goal.

Figure 11 shows the increase in utilization of services experienced by the Florida Medicaid program. Utilization grew as the new eligibility groups were added in 1987 through 1989. However, as huge numbers of new,

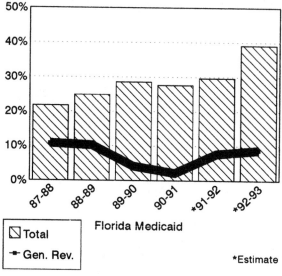

Combined Percentage Growth of Eligibles, Price and Utilization Percentage Growth in General Revenue

Florida Medicaid

☒ Total
➡ Gen. Rev.

*Estimate

Figure 12.

garden-variety AFDC recipients were added to the Medicaid rolls as a result of the worsening economy, overall utilization moderated and actually fell. The good news for fiscal analysts was that at least in the area of utilization, increases were less than growth in general revenue.

Summary of Medicaid Expenditure and Revenue Trends in Florida

All of these trends can be summarized in Figure 12. As can be seen, total Medicaid expenditures have greatly exceeded total general revenue growth in every year reported. While general revenue has grown on average at about 6.7 percent per year (range of 2 to 10 percent), Medicaid expenditures have grown on average 29 percent per year (range of 27 to 31.5 percent). Stated another way, Medicaid expenditures have grown more than four times faster than state revenues in the State of Florida over the past five years.

The net result is that state Medicaid agencies, and their various state legislatures, are facing a cost dynamic in which all of these forces—eligibility growth, inflation growth, and utilization growth—are both additive and mostly beyond their policy reach. Significant eligibility groups cannot be reduced: SSI income eligibility standards are federally determined; AFDC income levels cannot be dropped below 1988 standards per Medicare Catastrophic; and pregnant women, children to various ages, and Qualified Medicare Beneficiaries are all mandatory. Moreover, numbers of recipients are driven ever upward by a faltering national economy and by mandated "outreach."

Similarly, for the biggest portions of Medicaid spending—hospitals,

Florida Medicaid Appropriations
As a Percentage of Total State Budget

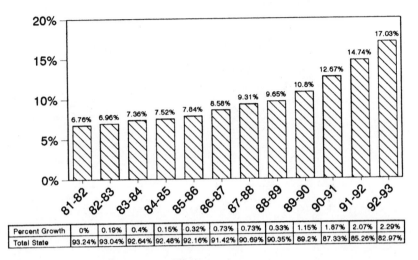

Percent Growth	0%	0.19%	0.4%	0.15%	0.32%	0.73%	0.73%	0.33%	1.15%	1.87%	2.07%	2.29%
Total State	93.24%	93.04%	92.64%	92.48%	92.16%	91.42%	90.69%	90.35%	89.2%	87.33%	85.26%	82.97%

◨ Medicaid

Figure 13.

nursing homes, and ICF/MRs—inflation cannot be driven down below certain Boren Amendment guarantees that now look like they must approximate full cost reimbursement. Physician prices are now being moved upward (including serious discussions of Medicare parity), and downward movement on prescription drug prices is forbidden (OBRA 1990). Even utilization, the least significant of the factors, is governed by "medically necessary" standards—putting additional burdens on the state to justify its service coverage on a case-by-case basis.

The results are predictable. As shown in Figure 13, in not a single year in the decade of the '80s and early into the 1990s has the Medicaid program accounted for an equal or smaller share of the overall state budget than the previous year. Instead, by increasing faster than general revenue, Medicaid is becoming an increasingly larger percentage of the total—more than doubling in Florida in ten years. From 6.8 percent of the total budget in 1981–82, the Medicaid percentage has increased to 17 percent—or almost one dollar in every six.

Even these figures, however, understate the prodigious shift in state priorities required to achieve this growth. In 1984–85, for instance, the Medicaid program accounted for 7.5 percent of all state spending and captured 9.9 percent of new general revenue—not a radical alteration in priorities. But by 1990–91, the program accounted for 12.7 percent of all state spending, but a whopping 39 percent of new general revenue. By 1991

171

New General Revenue

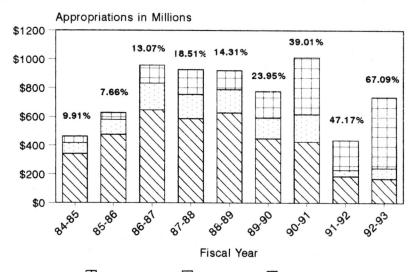

Figure 14.

and 1992 (years of marked economic downturns in revenue while eligibles skyrocketed), Medicaid consumed 47 and 67 percent of all new revenue respectively (see Figure 14).

Clearly, state legislators' hands are so tied by this one entitlement program that all other needs are being crowded out. Soon, given current trends, the state may be required to cut all other existing state programs to simply continue the Medicaid program at current levels! Additional enhancements, in terms of price, services, or new eligibility groups, will only exacerbate the problem.

IMPACT OF THE MEDICAID CHANGES ON ACCESS

More than a decade ago, Aaron Wildavsky, far better known as a political scientist than a health policy analyst, wrote a truly insightful article I believe was entitled "Doing Better, but Feeling Worse." I can hardly think of a more apt description of the state of the Medicaid program today. While we are clearly feeling ill about the enormous increases in expenditures, there are plenty of indicators that we are doing the right thing. Not all of these indicators of increased access can be measured with exact precision. But we do believe we are "doing better." Here are a few examples.

Indicator 1. Infant mortality rates are down, not just in Florida, but nationwide, as we had hoped. In Florida, for the first time in more than a

Infant Mortality Trends Rate Per 1000 Live Births

Year	Florida	United States
1960	29.7	26.0
1970	21.4	26.0
1980	14.5	12.6
1981	13.3	11.9
1982	12.8	11.5
1983	12.2	11.2
1984	10.8	10.8
1985	11.3	10.6
1986	11.0	10.4
1987	10.5	10.1
1988	10.6	9.9
1989	9.8	**9.7
1990	9.6	**9.1
1991	*8.9	Not Avail.

* Florida Vital Statistics Preliminary Final Data
** Provisional Data/Nat. Ctr. for Health Statistics

SOURCES:
FLORIDA VITAL STATISTICS
US STATISTICAL ABSTRACT
NAT. CENTER FOR HEALTH STATISTICS

Figure 15.

decade, we have performed better than the national average on infant mortality (see Figure 15).

Indicator 2. Provider access is up dramatically. As shown in Figure 16, physician services have grown the same as, or faster than, recipients in every year since we began our fee increase and provider responsiveness program (October 1987). In addition, as shown in Figure 17, the total number of providers has just about doubled—an increase of 10,000 physicians in four years.

Indicator 3. Our public health and MCH providers have dramatically increased their programs and access with the infusion of new Medicaid funds. In 1986, our statewide Improved Pregnancy Outcome (IPO) program saw about 40,000 pregnant women. Today, as a result of enormously increased Medicaid collections, it serves 80,000 persons without the need for an increase in the state general revenue that previously funded the program. Similarly, in 1991–92, after implementation of the EPSDT requirements of OBRA 1989, Medicaid paid for so many services that were not previously covered under the state plan that our crippled childrens' program (CMS) ran its first ever budget surplus. Traditionally, the program had terminated accepting new eligibles or contracting for new services three to five months before the end of the fiscal year, due to exhaustion of state general revenue funds.

Indicator 4. We know that hospital "boarder" babies in many parts of the state are virtually a phenomenon of the past, thanks to extensive in-home services, therapy programs, and other community services funded by OBRA 1989.

Indicator 5. We know that our traditional hospital partners in serving the poor and uninsured are doing far better than previously—despite still narrow financial margins. Public and teaching hospitals today rarely see an indigent pregnancy that is not paid for by Medicaid and have almost entirely stopped the financial hemorrhaging once seen in their neonatal intensive care units.

Medicaid Growth in Physician Services
Medicaid Growth in Eligibles

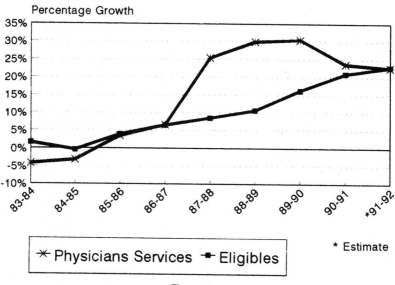

Figure 16.

Governmental hospitals, and particularly the top ten charity hospitals in Florida, have benefitted disproportionately by all the changes occasioned by state and federal law since 1986. Over half of all inpatient monies expended on the new eligibility groups have been concentrated in the ten percent of the hospital sector owned or operated by government entities. Over 80 percent of all new Medicaid hospital expenditures as a result of these expansions have gone to just the ten hospitals (out of more than 300) that provide over 80 percent of the charity care in the state. As a result— while overall hospital margins for the entire industry have declined rapidly with the advent of DRGs and other health system changes during this same time period—margins of the top ten charity hospitals in Florida have actually improved compared to 1987 lows. In fact, in two of the most recent three years, these top ten indigent care hospitals have recorded better average margins than the hospital industry as a whole (Figure 18).

Indicator 6. Managed care programs are growing at an even faster rate than the entire Medicaid program. HMO enrollment grew by 68 percent in just one year—from 95,000 to 160,000 between Fiscal Year 1990–91 and 1991–92 (see Figure 19). In addition, an experimental primary care case management program (MediPass) is projected to extend statewide in two years—with the enthusiastic support of organized medicine.

Indicator 7. Undoubtedly to the amazement of many providers and analysts familiar with state Medicaid programs of the 1970s and early 1980s,

Medicaid Provider Enrollment
Physicians and all Other Providers

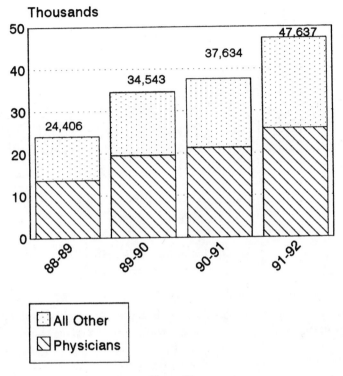

Figure 17.

we have begun to build systems of health care for poor people that work. Pregnancy outcomes in our IPO program are actually better than for the rest of the population. Our crippled children's programs are now being copied, or contracted with, by private industry and insurers. Both programs are primarily financed by Medicaid and operated by sister state agencies. Many providers find Medicaid payments faster and more reliable—if lesser in amount—than Medicare or private insurance. And chronically disabled children, AIDS patients, the elderly, and the developmentally disabled are treated more flexibly and appropriately by Medicaid than by Medicare or most private insurers.

LESSONS FOR THE FUTURE

Fundamental policy changes made to the Medicaid program since 1986 probably outweigh all changes made to the program in the previous 21 years since its inception. Rule and statute changes, interest group

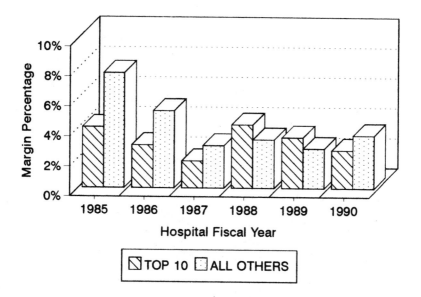

Margin Comparison
Top 10 Charity Hospitals vs. All Other Hospitals

Figure 18.

pressure, and incessant litigation have dramatically quickened the pace at all state Medicaid agencies. Amazingly, within the next year, Medicaid—the small 1965 afterthought to Medicare—will become the largest and most expensive of the nation's health care programs (federal and state expenditures combined). *What have we learned from these six years of Medicaid change?*

First, we can break the paradigm that has inextricably linked our health programs with cash assistance programs. However, we soon must go farther if we are to meet the health insurance needs of this country.

Second, we can set reasonable uniform standards for states to implement national programs, expect reasonable compliance, and at the same time retain considerable state flexibility.

Third, states can rather quickly adapt to new federal changes (if not within two months as sometimes mandated by Congress) and design and administer systems that are still responsive to their own needs and desires. In addition, the costs of these Medicaid claims processing and related administrative systems are far less than either Medicare or private insurance.

Fourth, in our urgency to expand the reach of federal aid through the Medicaid program, we can sometimes tip the scales too far. Not every worthwhile social work or educational service should be paid for on the health insurance/fee-for-service/freedom-of-choice paradigm that currently governs the Medicaid program. Other forms of federal aid may be needed in place of one with a built-in predilection to cost escalation—particularly in areas where need is

Florida Medicaid
Managed Health Care Growth

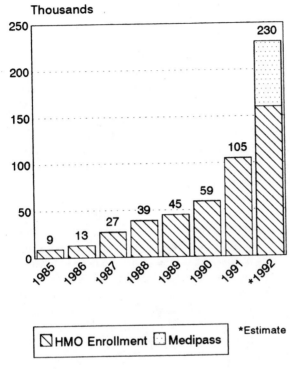

Thousands

Figure 19.

even less well-defined than medical care.

Fifth, we may have overdone it in our attempts to safeguard the economic future of traditional health care providers to the indigent. Recent federal changes to create disproportionate share payments for hospitals, and full cost reimbursement for community health centers, have greatly aided these providers. Nonetheless, by making such premium payments and arguing over guaranteed "market share" of Medicaid recipients, we are running a terrible danger of freezing in place an old system of health care just when there is a new willingness by many private providers and organizations to serve Medicaid patients.

Sixth, new forms of federal aid (and state regulation) are needed to assure that affordable health insurance is available to lower income workers and small business employees. Otherwise, we face the prospect that almost half of our population will be covered by the only other solution—Medicaid. This prospect is already the reality for the families of young pregnant mothers and their children. In Florida this year, more than 40 percent of all live births will occur to women on the Medicaid rolls. In some other states, the proportion is as high as two thirds.

Seventh, states simply cannot be expected to finance (on average) 45 percent of the cost of moving to national health insurance coverage for all. The current rates of growth for even a limited population are not sustainable for long—and are even less capable of supporting any dramatic expansion.

The citizens of this country need a guarantee of access to affordable health insurance coverage. But shuffling toward a national health insurance program by requiring the states to finance almost half of the cost, as we currently seem to be doing, seems certain to founder. The recent use of "provider taxes and donations" has greatly mitigated the effects of mandates and the faltering economy. But it has only delayed the need to grapple with the inevitable realization that states cannot finance the mounting bills of the Medicaid program and then have anything left over for any other human need, without radically changing (and increasing) their tax structures.

There is nothing inherently contradictory about having a national guarantee of access for affordable, quality health insurance and still having states involved in policy setting and administration. Indeed, that is the model of most other countries. As we continue to move toward national uniformity in the Medicaid program—a move well under way in terms of eligibility, adequacy of prices, and covered services—the federal government must begin buying out the additional costs of state governments. States should be required, however, to maintain their current financial effort, together with reasonable escalators for population (as opposed to recipient) growth and health care inflation.

Such an approach would place the additional costs for movement to a national health care program to the level of government most likely to have the means to pay for it. At the same time, it would retain considerable interest in each of the states in moderating health care inflation and in designing and supporting responsive, local systems of health care.

Finally, all of us who work in these Medicaid programs believe we have much to offer our citizens. In addition, we aspire for the day that each citizen of the United States can be assured of access to dignified, reasonably priced, quality health services—regardless of the number or name of the program. Hopefully, our experiences will help get us there a little faster.

SUMMARY

•

Summary of the Roundtable Discussion, July 21, 1992

KAREN DAVIS

The Kaiser Commission on the Future of Medicaid roundtable discussion and background papers focus on the growth in Medicaid costs, what factors are contributing to the growth, and the policy implications of the cost increases. The impact of the rising Medicaid costs on the availability of care for the poor is of particular concern.

The Commission background papers contained in this volume show that Medicaid historically has been a follower rather than a leader in health spending, growing at a slightly slower rate than private health care or Medicare spending. Starting in 1989, however, Medicaid departed dramatically from its prior patterns of increase, with spending more than doubling in the period from 1988 to 1992.

The recent upsurge in Medicaid spending reflects both the growth in the size of the population enrolled in Medicaid and increases in Medicaid spending per beneficiary owing to inflation, utilization, and Medicaid price increases beyond medical care price inflation. The roundtable discussion reviewed the growth in enrollment caused by federal legislation mandating expansions in Medicaid eligibility to cover more pregnant women and children and to supplement Medicare coverage for low-income elderly people. Federal mandates account for only a small part of the growth in Medicaid outlays. A portion of the enrollment increase reflects the recession's impact on expanding the numbers of people without employment-based insurance resulting in more low-income people poor enough to qualify for Medicaid benefits. The remaining enrollment growth reflects broader program participation in Aid to Families with Dependent Children (AFDC) and Medicaid among the disabled. In addition, there has been an increase in the disabled population enrolled in the federal Supplemental Security Income (SSI) program who are also eligible for Medicaid assistance.

Although there was general accord at the roundtable regarding the critical value of Medicaid coverage in increasing access to health care services for the low-income population, there was uncertainty regarding the adequacy of the coverage afforded to the low-income population by Medicaid. Some raised concerns about whether Medicaid beneficiaries are getting the services they require from the providers who are best able to furnish them and uncertainty about what Medicaid is really paying for. Given the growing pressure to limit resources for Medicaid-covered services, it is particularly critical to assure maximum value for dollars spent.

These reservations led some participants to touch upon their apprehensions over the potential impact of entitlement caps on federal and state spending, particularly on how such caps might affect the services offered and beneficiaries covered by Medicaid. Concern was expressed over the use of federal entitlement caps at a time when there has been growing reliance on Medicaid as the vehicle to expand health care coverage to the low-income population and provide protection to especially vulnerable populations, including the homeless, substance abusers, and people with AIDS. Entitlement caps are viewed as a crude policy instrument that could undermine the adequacy of Medicaid coverage and benefits.

It was noted that, in addition to enrollment growth, there has been a rise in the expenditures per beneficiary. Medical price inflation is, in part, responsible. Although Medicaid payments to providers have long been below those made by Medicare and the private sector, the program has not operated within a vacuum. It, too, has been affected by the unrestrained rate of growth in health care spending. Although Medicaid payment rates to providers are low relative to other payers, they cannot fall too low for fear of threatening access to care for program beneficiaries. Low Medicaid payments to physicians have been cited as a major contributor to the eroding rate of physician participation in Medicaid, resulting in reduced access. There is apprehension that the potential exists for hospitals and other providers also to become reluctant to accept Medicaid beneficiaries, further compromising access for the poor.

During this period, although payments to providers were lower than those of other payers, Medicaid spending accelerated far more rapidly than the rate of medical price inflation. This growth was a function of greater use of services and Medicaid price increases above levels needed to keep up with rising health care costs. In part, expenditure growth above inflation may be related to greater enrollment among sicker populations—such as those who are faced with the problems of AIDS or substance abuse—that further burden Medicaid as its stretches its funds to try to meet the society's changing needs. Not only is Medicaid serving as a social safety net, as illustrated by the background papers, changes in enrollment and eligibility policy to facilitate program participation now allow individuals to be enrolled in hospitals and at other providers at the very time they are using costly services. As a result, Medicaid's newly enrolled beneficiaries may carry higher service costs than beneficiaries historically enrolled in these categories because they are enrolling at the same time that they are using care.

The major factor, however, that appears to be driving increased outlays per beneficiary are Medicaid reimbursement levels. States have recently had to increase payments to providers, above the levels states deem appropriate for care within their budgets. This action is partially attributable to litigation under the Boren Amendment, a federal standard in the Medicaid statute for determining the "reasonableness" of payments to nursing homes and hospitals. In addition, concerns about assuring access to obstetricians and pediatricians as well as entities now referred to as Federally Qualified Health Centers led to a series of provider reimbursement reforms enacted in 1989 and 1990 that required states to increase payment levels. Although it was agreed that it still may be too soon to determine the influence of these reforms on Medicaid spending, it was acknowledged that this legislation would be a contributor to future spending increases.

Conference participants recognized that not all of the payment increases reflected reimbursement increases due to access concerns. Some, in fact, reflected state use of financing mechanisms to increase federal matching funds to support care for the uninsured, as well as to leverage state Medicaid contributions to finance expansions in coverage.

Legislatively, Medicaid payment rates cannot exceed Medicare rates except for payments to disproportionate share hospitals, those facilities providing a high volume of care to the poor and uninsured. Conference participants noted that disproportionate share payments have escalated dramatically and have been used to finance the care of the uninsured by many hospitals. The funds, in fact, represent substantial support to care of the uninsured.

States have aggressively sought out the use of other alternative financing techniques to increase federal revenues flowing to the states. These approaches used dollars raised by the states to leverage additional federal Medicaid matching funds. In the case of provider taxes and donations, the states either imposed a tax or required a donation from hospitals or nursing homes. This money, in turn, was used to leverage additional federal funds. In the care of intergovernmental transfers, funds contributed by local government were used to raise federal matching funds. Recent legislation is intended to stem these practices by limiting qualifying taxes and placing a ceiling on disproportionate share payments. Some observers commented that the states' increased use of these strategies to raise more federal dollars reflects the fiscal pressures that states face as they struggle with the increasing burdens of the reliance on Medicaid as a safety net program.

IMPLICATIONS

Over the course of the 1980s, federal grants-in-aid to the states fell dramatically. Federal policy eliminated or reduced funding for virtually all functions other than health and welfare. In this context, states shifted programs that were previously financed with state-only dollars to Medicaid. This practice, commonly referred to as Medicaid maximization, refinances existing programs with Medicaid dollars. Medicaid has thus become one of the only sources for support of many state-operated programs—mostly devoted to vulnerable populations.

Changes in federal budget policy that occurred in the mid-1980s further enhanced growth in Medicaid. While appropriated grant programs could only be increased at the expense of other "discretionary spending" or with new taxes, Medicaid and other entitlement programs were exempted from budgetary ceilings. As a result, Medicaid became virtually the only means for pursuing improvements in the health-related safety net. Increasingly, budget policy, not health policy, has determined federal actions and enhanced Medicaid's role.

In sum, from the background papers and the discussion, there was general agreement on the factors underlying the spending growth. Enrollment growth has been an important contributor to the increase in Medicaid spending, but cost increases in prices paid for service and service use were equally important. Further analysis of the role of each of these contributing factors was viewed as an essential part of future analytic efforts to understand the spending trends in this program.

The participants agreed that, in the absence of national health reform, the problems Medicaid is confronting are not likely to subside in the near future. Coverage expansions are continuing to be phased-in through the year 2001, health care inflation continues to grow at an unrestrained rate, and 37 million Americans are uninsured. In addition, Medicaid is increasingly becoming a source of financing for traditionally non-medical spending such as social services, education, and care of the developmentally disabled. At the same time, states are finding themselves unable or unwilling to generate the additional revenues needed to finance their share of Medicaid and the federal government is facing the largest deficit in history.

The participants concluded that Medicaid's problems cannot be resolved without fundamental reform of the health care financing and delivery system for all Americans. To begin to resolve the problems facing the Medicaid program and health care for the low-income population, many questions need to be answered. Who has responsibility to pay for health care of the poor? Should the states continue to share the costs, and if so at what level? Should Medicaid be federalized? Should there be separate programs for acute and long-term care? Should Medicaid be abolished altogether and replaced with a universal program or with a new, nationally uniform program for the poor? How do we design health care delivery systems to best serve the low-income population? What is the most effective way to control costs in the health system overall, without jeopardizing access to quality care for low-income people? The participants of the discussion viewed this agenda of issues as integral to designing an adequate system to finance care to the low-income and vulnerable populations. The Commission looks forward to the challenge embodied in attempting to address these critical issues.

EPILOGUE

•

The Kaiser Commission on the Future of Medicaid: Findings and Implications

DIANE ROWLAND AND
ALINA SALGANICOFF

Unanswered questions raised by the previous chapters and the roundtable discussion underscored the need for further examination of the contributions of multiple components of the unprecedented rise in Medicaid spending. The Commission subsequently sponsored research by the Urban Institute to provide additional analysis to disaggregate the contribution of enrollment growth, medical price inflation, and increased service intensity to the overall increase in Medicaid spending from 1988 to 1991. The findings of the research and the Commission's conclusions are presented in the Kaiser Commission on the Future of Medicaid's report, *The Medicaid Cost Explosion: Causes and Consequences,* and are highlighted in this chapter.

FINDINGS

From 1988 to 1991, national spending on Medicaid services grew $37.0 billion, from $51.6 billion to $88.6 billion. The Commission's findings indicate that this growth is attributable to three major influences: increases in enrollment, growth in medical price inflation, and increases in expenditures per person served by the program. Each accounts for roughly one third of the expenditure growth. A small share of the growth is also attributable to spending on Medicare premiums and payments to health maintenance organizations.

Growth in Medicaid enrollment accounted for 34 percent of the increase in expenditures from 1988 to 1991. During this period, enrollment grew from 22.2 million to 27.0 million individuals, resulting in an additional 4.8 million beneficiaries. Half of the new Medicaid beneficiaries were the pregnant women and children covered as a result of state expansions that are driven, in part, by federal requirements to broaden coverage for this population. Although they represent the bulk of new enrollees, the costs associated with the coverage of this group account for only 11 percent of total growth in that period. This finding stands in sharp contrast to the common perception that federal mandates expanding coverage for pregnant women and children have largely been responsible for the cost explosion. In fact, enrollment increases in traditional Medicaid populations such as AFDC families and the aged and disabled represent the other half of the new enrollees and account for nearly one fourth of total expenditure growth. This reflects the higher costs associated with the acute and long-term care services for disabled and elderly beneficiaries.

Medical price inflation was responsible for 31 percent of the expenditure growth during the 1988-to-1991 period. This factor is outside of Medicaid's control and underscores the fact that Medicaid purchases care for its beneficiaries in the overall health care marketplace. Medicaid expenditures cannot be addressed in isolation from the rest of the health care system.

Increase in spending per beneficiary represents 28 percent of the total growth. It reflects the influences of growing demand for services from sicker populations, increased payment to providers as a result of litigation and legislation, and increases in state use of alternative financing systems to bring in federal dollars.

IMPLICATIONS

The recent dramatic escalation in Medicaid costs is understandably a cause of concern. However, analysis of its components and its causes reveals that, for the most part, cost increases reflect a program doing its job. Medicaid's cost increases indicate that dependence on its role as the nation's health care safety net, medical price inflation, and the realignment of federal/state financing responsibilities creates the pressures that propel higher spending. Corrective action requires that we focus broadly on these problems, rather than narrowly on Medicaid costs, in order to protect effectively the nation's poor and vulnerable at an acceptable cost.

Foremost evidence of this conclusion is that more than a third of recent spending growth reflects Medicaid's expansion to cover growing numbers of poor and vulnerable Americans—the very purpose for which it was established. Contrary to conventional wisdom, only a small proportion of cost growth comes from newly enrolled pregnant women and children, for whom state and federal governments have deemed coverage essential. These legislatively mandated expansions are providing needed coverage to millions, but their per capita costs are relatively small. Expanded enrollment among far smaller numbers of persons with disabilities impose much greater per capita costs, which, at this time, only Medicaid is willing to bear. It is spending for these groups that dominates the enrollment-related expenditure increases in Medicaid.

Further evidence of the costs of securing Medicaid as a financing source of vulnerable populations is health care inflation as a contributor to Medicaid costs. Like all other payers of health care, Medicaid struggles with meeting its responsibilities in the face of escalating health care prices. To ignore health cost inflation would worsen access to the very protection Medicaid aims to provide. Nearly one third of the recent cost explosion can be explained simply in terms of preserving that protection, by keeping payment increases at least in line with increases in the cost of health services nationwide. Clearly, any national curb on health care price increases will benefit Medicaid.

Use and payment increases above inflation are harder to characterize. This third of the recent cost explosion reflects a variety of factors, including more costly service to sicker populations, enhanced services for children, higher payment levels for providers attributable to litigation, Medicaid maximization, and alternative financing mechanisms by states to increase federal matching payments.

The recent legislation limiting state ability to draw federal Medicaid matching funds through provider taxes and donations will place even greater budgetary pressure on state Medicaid programs and may bring the states to the brink of fiscal crisis. This action, coupled with the trend in decreasing federal grants-in-aid to the states for other social welfare programs, increases the fiscal pressure states face in providing health coverage to vulnerable populations. Given the economic climate and the growing need for health care assistance, states are faced with limited choices in operating their Medicaid programs. Constrained by eligibility and benefit requirements, and the need to provide adequate payment to safeguard access, states are left with few alternatives. If they are unable to generate sufficient general revenues, they may be forced to make sharp program cutbacks. Reliance on Medicaid as the vehicle to expand coverage and services to the poor, coupled with restraints on state revenue sources that can be matched by the federal government, may place states in an untenable situation.

These findings lead the Commission to conclude that efforts to focus on or resolve a "Medicaid crisis"—viewed in isolation—are a mistake. Rather, the real crisis is the growing need for health insurance coverage for the poor and disabled; unrestrained health care costs; and fiscal tension between state and federal governments, rather than effectively shared responsibility. Only an examination of these broader problems, and the most effective role of a safety net within them, can ensure adequate protection for the nation's poor and vulnerable.

NEXT STEPS

The Commission is continuing to work toward fulfilling its mandate to provide independent analysis and information on health care issues impacting our nation's low-income and vulnerable population and thus contribute to the public debate on health care reform. In response to the Commission's conclusions that the problems that are afflicting Medicaid are systemic in nature, the subsequent activities that have been undertaken have focused on both the delivery system and the special needs of the low-income population. Presently, the Commission is in the process of examining health care service and delivery issues affecting the low-income population and the providers that serve them. Specifically, they will be examining the health status of low-income people, the role of safety net providers, how the low-income population uses the existing delivery system, and the implications of managed care for the low-income population. It is our hope that the efforts of the Commission will culminate in a Commission report on access and service delivery to the low-income population, as well as a volume, such as this, containing the access and service delivery background papers sponsored by the Commission.

APPENDIX A
•

Principal Federal
Medicaid Legislative Reforms
1981–1991

SARA ROSENBAUM

The following five tables set forth the principal Medicaid reforms enacted between 1981 and 1991. Over this time period literally hundreds of revisions in Medicaid were adopted. The information in the tables provides a summary of the most significant changes enacted to date.

The amendments described in the tables were enacted for a wide variety of reasons. Some were adopted in order to curtail federal and state Medicaid expenditures on certain populations or certain health care benefits or to reduce state spending flexibility. Others were enacted in order to expand coverage and benefits. Still others were adopted to increase states' flexibility in administering their programs or to reduce federal financial participation in states' Medicaid programs.

The reforms presented in these tables represent significant departures from prior law and have (or can be expected to have) a major impact on the way in which the program functions for beneficiaries, providers, and states. Some of the changes were identified by the Congressional Budget Office and the Office of Management and Budget as financially significant at the time of enactment, but others (including some very important changes) were envisioned as costing relatively little. Still others were probably given cost estimates that will prove to be far too high.

Where a change is identified as having either a plus or minus cost impact, this represents an estimate of its practical effects, rather than the formal cost estimate calculated by either federal budget office. For example, in 1990 the OMB identified mandated outstationed enrollment for pregnant women and children as having no, or minimal, budget impact. In practice, however, outstationing appears to have a major effect on the proportion of Medicaid-enrolled eligible pregnant women and children. Therefore, it can be expected to increase overall program costs as a practical matter.

The tables are divided into five separate sets:

- eligibility-related changes,

- changes in benefits,

- changes affecting provider reimbursement,

- changes affecting state administration, and

- changes affecting federal financial participation.

Each set describes the principal changes enacted each year. Not reflected in the tables are all of the technical and "perfecting" revisions to already enacted legislation. Nor are the scores of demonstration authorities contained in each year's legislation included. A separate study of the demonstrations under Medicaid that have been authorized over the past 10 years, along with information on results achieved, probably would be of great value.

Also not shown on these tables are all of the changes in related programs [such as Aid to Families with Dependent Children (AFDC) and Supplemental Security Income (SSI)] that affect Medicaid spending. However, some of the most important revisions in cash welfare programs are shown because of their sizable impact on the nature and scope of state Medicaid programs. To be truly complete in their depiction of changing federal program policy on Medicaid coverage and costs, these tables would incorporate not only every change in Medicaid enacted since 1981, but every change in every federal law that could reasonably be expected to affect Medicaid eligibility, coverage, and expenditure levels. These federal laws include, but are not limited to, AFDC, SSI, Child Support Enforcement, Social Security Old Age Survivors and Disability Insurance, Medicare, Child Welfare and Adoption Assistance, and Unemployment Compensation.

Table 1. Medicaid Eligibility.

Type of Reform	Act and Year of Reform	Program Impact Assessment
Limitation on AFDC earned income disregards: MANDATORY.	§2301, P.L. 97–35, Omnibus Budget Reconciliation Act (OBRA) of 1981	*Restricts eligibility:* Limits AFDC (and therefore Medicaid eligibility for working AFDC recipient families) by increasing amount of countable income credited against applicants and beneficiaries with earnings. Limitations mean that families may keep less earned income and still qualify for AFDC and Medicaid.

Table 1. Medicaid Eligibility. (continued)

Type of Reform	Act and Year of Reform	Program Impact Assessment
150 percent "cap" on amount by which applicants' gross family income can exceed the AFDC standard of need: MANDATORY.	§2303, P.L. 97–35, OBRA 1981	*Restricts eligibility:* Limits eligibility for AFDC and Medicaid by placing upper limits on total income applicants may have and still apply for or receive AFDC and Medicaid. Even if countable income falls below AFDC/Medicaid eligibility level, families can be disqualified under gross income test.
Prohibition against pro-rating lump sum payments: MANDATORY.	§2304, P.L. 97–35, OBRA 1981	*Restricts eligibility:* Persons receiving lump sum payments must declare all income (such as child support arrearages) in month in which it is received, rather than allocating it over several months in order to retain AFDC and Medicaid eligibility.
Deeming step-parent income: MANDATORY.	§2306, P.L. 97–35, OBRA 1981	*Restricts eligibility:* Attributes additional countable income to children living with families and applying for or receiving AFDC and Medicaid. Note: subsequent court decisions struck down application of this change to Medicaid-only applicants, but it is unclear how many persons, once denied AFDC and Medicaid, nonetheless applied for Medicaid for their children.

Table 1. Medicaid Eligibility. (continued)

Type of Reform	Act and Year of Reform	Program Impact Assessment
AFDC maximum age limited to age 19: MANDATORY.	§2311, P.L. 97–35, OBRA 1981	*Restricts eligibility:* age limit at 19 for receipt of both AFDC and Medicaid.
Elimination of AFDC unborn child program and limitation of AFDC benefits to final three months of pregnancy: MANDATORY.	§2312, P.L. 97–35, OBRA 1981	*Restricts eligibility:* Eliminates AFDC coverage for unborn children. Permits pregnant women to receive AFDC only during final three months of pregnancy but retains Medicaid from time pregnancy is verified. Note: while states could continue to grant Medicaid benefits, lack of clarifying rules caused many states to discontinue both.
Limitations on AFDC eligibility for unemployed families: MANDATORY.	§2313, P.L. 97–35, OBRA 1981	*Restricts eligibility:* AFDC-UP limited to families whose *principal* wage earner is unemployed, even if income loss from "secondary" unemployed wage earner brings gross and countable income below qualifying levels.
Retrospective budgeting and monthly reporting: MANDATORY.	§2315, P.L. 97–35, OBRA 1981	*Restricts eligibility:* Limits AFDC and Medicaid eligibility to persons whose past income falls below qualifying levels, even if current monthly income is low enough to qualify for benefits. Eligibility also restricted to persons who comply with monthly reporting requirements regarding changes in

Table 1. Medicaid Eligibility. (continued)

Type of Reform	Act and Year of Reform	Program Impact Assessment
		income, family composition, and living arrangements.
Elimination of AFDC payments under $10.00: MANDATORY.	§2316, P.L. 97–35, OBRA 1981	*Restricts eligibility:* Eliminates AFDC for persons with small monthly checks. While Medicaid termination not mandatory, related nature of the decision means loss of both program benefits.
Elimination of AFDC benefits for undocumented persons: MANDATORY.	§2318, P.L. 97–35, OBRA 1981	*Restricts AFDC eligibility, but no direct impact on Medicaid:* Denial of AFDC for persons who are not citizens or lawfully admitted for permanent United States residence or otherwise residing in the U.S. under color of law. Undocumented persons may still apply for Medicaid until 1986 (see discussion infra).
Retrospective budgeting for SSI applicants and recipients: MANDATORY.	§12776, P.L. 97–35, OBRA 1981	*Restricts eligibility:* Restricts SSI and Medicaid eligibility to persons who can qualify for assistance on the, basis of prior month's income.
Elimination of medically needy "comparability" requirements: OPTIONAL.	§2171, P.L. 97–35, OBRA 1981	*Both restricts and expands coverage:* Permits states with medically needy programs to limit coverage to pregnant women and ambulatory services for children under age 18. While some states may have

Table 1. Medicaid Eligibility. (continued)

Type of Reform	Act and Year of Reform	Program Impact Assessment
		reduced coverage, others added limited medically needy programs using new authority. Also permits states to use more restrictive eligibility levels for the medically needy than those used under the most closely related cash assistance program. Note: this change led to repeated amendments to clarify that states still retained the option to set more liberal standards and methodologies for Medicaid beneficiaries not receiving cash assistance.
Flexibility in coverage of children ages 19–21: OPTIONAL.	§2172, P.L. 97–35, OBRA 1981	*Restricts eligibility:* Permits states to terminate Medicaid coverage when child reaches age 19. States may continue, at their option, to cover some or all children ages 19–21. Note: Medicaid thus separated from AFDC, where termination became mandatory by age 19 under OBRA 1981.
Home care for disabled children: OPTIONAL.	§134, P.L. 97–248, Tax Equity and Fiscal Responsibility Act (TEFRA) of 1982	*Expands eligibility:* Permits coverage of children who otherwise would be eligible only as institutional recipients of SSI, so long as home care costs do not exceed estimated institutional costs.

Table 1. Medicaid Eligibility. (continued)

Type of Reform	Act and Year of Reform	Program Impact Assessment
Pregnant women added as separate class of Medicaid beneficiaries: OPTIONAL.	§137, P.L. 97–248, TEFRA 1982	*No cost impact:* However, represents first time that pregnant women are classified as eligible in their own right, as an independent eligibility category. Note: other optional coverage categories also expressly listed in the statute in 1982. These categories had previously existed by statutory implication and by rule.
Coverage of "qualified" children and pregnant women: MANDATORY.	§2361, P.L. 98–369, Deficit Reduction Act (DEFRA) of 1984	*Expands Eligibility:* Mandates coverage of "qualified" children (born after September 30, 1983, and under age 5, whose family incomes fall below state AFDC payment levels) and "qualified" pregnant women (who would be eligible for AFDC or for AFDC-UP if their children were born and living with them). Note: "qualified" women's and children's financial eligibility standards equal AFDC standards (approximately 40 percent of the federal poverty level).
Increase in AFDC "gross income" test: MANDATORY.	§2621, 2625, P.L. 98–369, DEFRA 1984	*Expands eligibility:* Raises from 150% to 185% the upper limit on gross family income for AFDC and Medicaid.
Extended eligibility for 9 months for certain employed families: MANDATORY.	§2374, P.L. 98–369, DEFRA 1984	*Expands eligibility:* Provides 9 months of additional coverage for persons losing AFDC

Table 1. Medicaid Eligibility. (continued)

Type of Reform	Act and Year of Reform	Program Impact Assessment
		and Medicaid benefits as a result of increased countable income from earnings as a result of the termination of certain earned income disregards.
Automatic coverage of newborns: MANDATORY.	§2368, P.L. 98–369, DEFRA 1984	*Expands eligibility:* Coverage for one year provided automatically to infants born to women receiving Medicaid so long as they continue to reside with their mothers and so long as their mothers remain eligible for Medicaid. (Note: in 1987 the statute was again amended to require states to permit mothers to use their medical assistance I.D. numbers to purchase care for their infants pending the arrival of the infants' cards).
Assignment of right to medical support: MANDATORY.	§2367, P.L. 98–369, DEFRA 1984	*Restricts eligibility:* Coverage limited to persons who agree to disclose all responsible third parties and assign right to medical support as condition of eligibility.
Extended Medicaid coverage for persons losing benefits because of increased child support: MANDATORY.	§303, P.L. 98–397, Child Support Enforcement Amendments of 1984	*Expands eligibility:* Coverage extended for 4 months for caretakers and children losing AFDC and Medicaid coverage because of increased child support collections.
Coverage of all pregnant women qualifying for AFDC on the basis of financial	§9501, P.L. 99–272, Consolidated Omnibus Budget Reconciliation	*Expands eligibility:* "Perfecting" amendment to "qualified" pregnant

Table 1. Medicaid Eligibility. (continued)

Type of Reform	Act and Year of Reform	Program Impact Assessment
criteria: MANDATORY. Immediate coverage of all "qualified" children. under age 5: MANDATORY	Act (COBRA) of 1985	women amendment in DEFRA, which extends coverage to all women whose children, if born, would be entitled to Medicaid as qualified children, thereby adding pregnant women in two-parent employed families. Also speeds up phased-in coverage of "qualified" children.
Post-partum eligibility for pregnant women: MANDATORY.	§9501, P.L. 99–272, COBRA 1985	*Expands eligibility:* Requires states to extend Medicaid for 60 post-partum days to women who received Medicaid while pregnant and who would otherwise lose coverage once their child was born.
Coverage of certain foster care and adoptive children: OPTIONAL.	§9511, P.L. 99–272, COBRA 1985	*Expands eligibility:* Permits states to extend Medicaid to certain children in state-funded foster care and adoptive arrangements, using the more generous eligibility standards normally applicable only to children in federally funded adoptive and foster care placements.
Preservation of Medicaid for certain widows and widowers: MANDATORY.	§12202, P.L. 99–272, COBRA 1985	*Expands eligibility:* Restores Medicaid to certain widows and widowers losing SSI and Medicaid because of changes in OASDI actuarial methodologies.
Medicaid eligibility extended to otherwise Medicaid-eligible	§201, P.L. 99–473, Immigration Reform and Control Act, 1986	*Expands eligibility:* Extends Medicaid to persons only temporarily

Table 1. Medicaid Eligibility. (continued)

Type of Reform	Act and Year of Reform	Program Impact Assessment
temporary resident aliens who are pregnant women, children, persons with emergency medical conditions,or elderly and disabled persons: MANDATORY.		(as opposed to permanently) residing under color of law who have been granted "amnesty" under the 1986 Immigration amendments. Coverage restricted to otherwise eligible pregnant women, children, and persons with medical emergencies or recipients of SSI.
Disqualification of applicants and recipients in the event of certain "qualifying trusts": MANDATORY.	§9506, P.L. 99–509, OBRA 1986	*Restricts eligibility:* Disqualifies from Medicaid certain persons who shield income and assets in so-called Medicaid "qualifying trusts."
Coverage of "poverty level" pregnant women and children: OPTIONAL.	§9401, P.L. 99–509, OBRA 1986	*Expands eligibility:* Permits states at their option to extend Medicaid to pregnant women, infants, and children under age 5 (phased in on a year-by-year basis) with family income below 100 percent of the federal poverty level. States permitted to disregard resources at their option.
Presumptive (i.e., temporary) eligibility for pregnant women for ambulatory Medicaid services: OPTIONAL. Continuous coverage for pregnant women: OPTIONAL	§9407, P.L. 99–509, OBRA 1986	*Expands eligibility:* Permits states at their option to extend temporary coverage for pregnant women who are initially presumed eligible for full coverage. Eligibility determined at health centers, Title-V assisted clinics, WIC agencies, and other

Table 1. Medicaid Eligibility. (continued)

Type of Reform	Act and Year of Reform	Program Impact Assessment
		maternal and child health service sites. Enrollment assistance provided on-site, along with temporary coverage. States also permitted to provide continuous coverage for pregnant women from the time Medicaid eligibility is granted through the post-partum period, regardless of changes in family income.
Coverage of qualified severely impaired persons: MANDATORY.	§9404, P.L. 99–509, OBRA 1986	*Expands eligibility:* Requires Medicaid coverage of persons enrolled in SSI who lose SSI because of earnings, who need continued Medicaid coverage to be able to continue working, and whose earnings are insufficient to replace the value of lost SSI, Medicaid, and Title XX benefits.
Payment for aliens: MANDATORY.	§9406, P.L. 99–509, OBRA 1986	*Restricts eligibility:* Eliminates coverage for persons who are not citizens, aliens lawfully admitted for permanent residents, temporary residents, or otherwise permanently residing under "color of law."
Coverage of poor Medicare beneficiaries for full Medicaid benefits: OPTIONAL.	§9402, P.L. 99–509, OBRA 1986	*Expands eligibility:* Permits states to cover elderly and disabled Medicare beneficiaries with family incomes below 100 percent of the federal poverty level and

Table 1. Medicaid Eligibility. (continued)

Type of Reform	Act and Year of Reform	Program Impact Assessment
		with assets that do not exceed federal standards.
Coverage of poor Medicare beneficiaries for Medicare costsharing: OPTIONAL.	§9403, P.L. 99–509, OBRA 1986	*Expands eligibility:* Permits states to extend Medicaid coverage of Medicare costsharing requirements (e.g., premiums, deductibles, and coinsurance) to elderly and disabled Medicare beneficiaries with family income below the federal poverty level and resources that do not exceed federally established levels.
Coverage of pregnant women and infants with family incomes up to 185 percent of the federal poverty level: OPTIONAL.	§4101, P.L. 100–203, OBRA 1987	*Expands eligibility:* Allows states to cover all pregnant women and infants with family incomes under 185 percent of poverty.
Mandatory coverage of all qualified children born after September 30, 1983, who have attained age 5 but who are under age 8 and optional coverage of poverty-level children up to age 8: MANDATORY AND OPTIONAL.	§4101, P.L. 100–203, OBRA 1987	*Expands eligibility:* Continues 1984 mandate to cover all qualified children, which originally ceased at age 5. Also allows states to cover poverty-level children up to age 8.
Extension of Medicaid coverage for 12 months for certain families following loss of AFDC due to increased actual or countable earnings: MANDATORY.	§303, P.L. 100–485, Family Support Act of 1988	*Expands eligibility:* Mandates 12 months of Medicaid coverage for families losing AFDC benefits as a result of increased actual or countable family earnings, if the family received AFDC during 3 of the preceding 6 months prior to termination.

Table 1. Medicaid Eligibility. (continued)

Type of Reform	Act and Year of Reform	Program Impact Assessment
Medical assistance for two-parent unemployed families: MANDATORY.	§401, P.L. 100–485, Family Support Act of 1988	*Expands eligibility:* Mandates Medicaid/ unemployed parent coverage for families meeting the AFDC-UP eligibility test, even if state has elected not to extend full AFDC-UP benefits.
Increase in earned income and child care disregards for working families receiving AFDC: MANDATORY.	§402, P.L. 100–485, Family Support Act of 1988	*Expands eligibility:* Liberalizes rules for treatment of earned income for AFDC and Medicaid purposes.
Disregard of advance earned income tax credit payments to working AFDC families: MANDATORY.	§402, P.L. 100–485, Family Support Act of 1988	*Expands eligibility:* Liberalizes rules for retention of family income while still qualifying for AFDC and Medicaid.
Coverage of pregnant women and infants with family incomes below 100 percent of the federal poverty level: MANDATORY.	§302, P.L. 100–360, Medicare Catastrophic Coverage Act (MCCA) of 1988	*Expands eligibility:* Mandates coverage of poverty-level pregnant women and infants whose coverage was made optional in 1986.
Mandatory coverage of Medicare premiums, deductibles, and coinsurance for poor Medicare beneficiaries, including beneficiaries enrolled in both Medicare and Medicaid: MANDATORY.	§301, P.L. 100–360, MCCA 1988; §8434(a), P.L. 100–647, Tax Technical and Miscellaneous Revenue Act of 1988	*Expands eligibility:* Mandates coverage of Medicare premiums, coinsurance, and deductibles for low-income beneficiaries, which was made optional in 1986. Note: mandatory eligibility standard subsequently raised to 120 percent of poverty for part B premiums only.
Protection of incomes and resources of couples for maintenance	§303, P.L. 100–360, MCCA 1988	*Expands eligibility:* Establishes new protected income and

Table 1. Medicaid Eligibility. (continued)

Type of Reform	Act and Year of Reform	Program Impact Assessment
of community spouse: MANDATORY.		resource levels for spouses of Medicaid recipients institution-alized in long-term care facilities to provide greater levels of financial support to non-institution-alized community spouses. Income level set at a minimum of 150% of monthly federal poverty level, not to exceed $1500 (indexed for CPI). Resource levels set at between $12,000 and $60,000 (indexed for CPI).
Coverage of poverty-level pregnant women and children born after September 30, 1983, and under age 6: MANDATORY.	§6401, P.L. 101–239, OBRA 1989	*Expands eligibility:* Mandates coverage of all pregnant women, infants, and children under age 6 (born after September 30, 1983) with family incomes below 133 percent of poverty. Increases mandated coverage levels for pregnant women and infants established under MCCA.
Mandated coverage of all children born after September 30, 1983, who have attained age 6 but not age 19, with family incomes below 100 percent of the federal poverty level: MANDATORY.	§4601, P.L 101–508, OBRA 1990	*Expands eligibility:* Extends mandatory coverage to all poor children under age 19, phased in on a year-by-year basis, beginning with children born after September 30, 1983.
Continuous benefits throughout pregnancy and age 1: MANDATORY.	§4603, P.L. 101–508. OBRA 1990	*Expands eligibility:* Mandates previous option first enacted in 1986 to provide

Table 1. Medicaid Eligibility. (continued)

Type of Reform	Act and Year of Reform	Program Impact Assessment
		continuous coverage to all pregnant women from the time that pregnancy is verified through the end of the post-partum period. Also provides that infants born to Medicaid women remain eligible through first year of life, without reapplication, even if mothers lose their own Medicaid coverage after post-partum period, so long as infant resides with its mother and mother would continue to be eligible for Medicaid if pregnant.
Revision of Medicaid spend-down program: OPTIONAL.	§4723, P.L. 101–508, OBRA 1990	*Expands eligibility:* Permits states at their option to allow spend-down applicants to pay anticipated incurred expenses in the form of prospective monthly payments rather than witholding coverage until the spend-down obligation has been actually incurred.
Liberalization of medically needy income standard for single persons: OPTIONAL.	§4718, P.L. 101–508, OBRA 1990	*Expands eligibility:* Permits certain states to use AFDC payment levels for a family of two to determine medically needy eligibility for a single person.

Table 2. Benefit Reforms.

Type of Reform	Act and Year of Reform	Program Impact Assessment
Pregnancy-related benefits: OPTIONAL.	§9501, P.L. 99-272 COBRA 1985	*Expands benefits:* Permits states to provide additional benefits to pregnant women not otherwise covered for Medicaid beneficiaries.
Habilitation services for persons discharged from institutional placements: OPTIONAL.	§9502, P.L. 99–272, COBRA 1985	*Expands benefits:* Permits states to cover broadly defined habilitation services to persons discharged from long-term care settings and participating in home- and community-based care waiver programs authorized in 1981.
Expanded home- and community-based services: OPTIONAL.	§9502, P.L. 99–272, COBRA 1985	*Expands benefits:* Permits states to furnish waivered home- and community-based benefits whose actual costs exceed estimated institutional care costs.
Coverage of hospice services: OPTIONAL.	§9505, P.L. 99–272, COBRA 1985	*Expands benefits:* Permits states to extend hospice coverage to beneficiaries. Hospice benefits are defined as services furnished to the terminally ill by a hospice program under a written treatment plan. Services include nursing care; physical, occupational, and speech therapy; medical social services; physicians' services; short-term inpatient care; and other services.
Organ transplants: OPTIONAL.	§9507, P.L. 99–272, COBRA 1985	*Restricts benefits:* Permits states to delete coverage of medically necessary, non-experimental organ transplants.

Table 2. Benefit Reforms (continued).

Type of Reform	Act and Year of Reform	Program Impact Assessment
Case management: OPTIONAL.	§9411, P.L. 99–272, COBRA 1985	*Expands benefits:* Permits states to extend targeted case management services to some or all portions of the Medicaid patient population as an optional Medicaid service.
Services for persons with AIDS: OPTIONAL.	§9411, P.L. 99–509, OBRA 1986	*Expands benefits:* Permits states to extend community-based care to persons with AIDS who otherwise would receive coverage in institutions.
Services for persons with mental illness: OPTIONAL.	§9412, P.L. 99–509, OBRA 1986	*Expands benefits:* Permits states to extend home and community care to persons with mental illness who otherwise would receive care in institutional settings.
Federally qualified health centers: MANDATORY.	§6404, P.L. 101–234, OBRA 1989	*Expands benefits:* Requires states to cover certain federally qualified health center services, defined as physician, mid-level, psychology and social work, and ancillary services offered by federally qualified health centers (FQHCs). FQHCs include all federally funded community and migrant health centers and homeless health care programs as well as entities meeting those requirements.
Expansion of nursing facility services and preadmission screening and resident review	100–203, OBRA 1987 §9516, P.L. 99–272, COBRA 1985; §4211, P.L.	*Expands benefits:* Increases state responsibilities to develop comprehensive and

Table 2. Benefit Reforms (continued).

Type of Reform	Act and Year of Reform	Program Impact Assessment
(PASSAR) activities: MANDATORY.		appropriate treatment programs for nursing home residents and persons with mental illness and mental retardation.
Early and Periodic Screening Diagnosis and Treatment: MANDATORY.	§6403, P.L. 101–239, OBRA 1989	*Expands benefits:* Amends the EPSDT program originally added to the statute in 1967 as a special benefit package for all children under age 21 enrolled in Medicaid. Amendments continue prior requirement that states cover medically appropriate periodic medical, dental, vision, and hearing exams as well as vision, dental and hearing care and other care and services covered under the state plan. Adds as new requirements: exams whenever a problem is suspected, as well as all medically necessary care recognized under the federal definition of medical assistance (§1905(a) of the Social Security Act) regardless of whether such services are offered to persons over age 21. Amount, scope, and duration limits must be consistent with the preventive purposes of EPSDT and medical necessity standards.

Table 2. Benefit Reforms (continued).

Type of Reform	Act and Year of Reform	Program Impact Assessment
Coverage of nurse practitioner services: MANDATORY.	§6405, P.L. 101–239, OBRA 1989	*Expands benefits:* Requires states to cover pediatric nurse practitioner services to maximum extent to which such services are legally authorized under state law.
Home- and community-based care for functionally disabled elderly individuals: OPTIONAL.	§4711, P.L. 101–508, OBRA 1990	*Expands benefits:* Permits states to offer as an optional Medicaid benefit home- and community-based services to functionally disabled elderly persons who receive SSI or who are medically needy, with prior home and community-based waiver patients grandfathered into new optional programs. Permits coverage for medically needy persons based on projected income and expenses, establishes service, treatment plan, and provider require-ments, and sets out an aggregate per quarter expenditure cap. Also places upper federal limit on amount of funds made available for this new benefit.
Community-supported living arrangements: OPTIONAL.	§4711, P.L. 101–508, OBRA 1990	*Expands Services:* Permits states to establish community supported living arrange-ment programs for developmentally disabled individuals, with no less

Table 2. Benefit Reforms (continued).

Type of Reform	Act and Year of Reform	Program Impact Assessment
		than two and no more than eight states permitted to participate. Eligible individuals are those who meet federal developmental disability requirements and who live in their own home or in an apartment, family home, or rental unit furnished in a community-supported living arrangement. Annual federal expenditure ceilings set.
Payment of health insurance premiums where cost effective: MANDATORY.	§§4402 and 4713, P.L. 101–508, OBRA 1990	*Potentially Reduces costs:* Requires states to pay health insurance premiums (including COBRA premiums, if applicable) where cost effective and pay other cost-sharing for benficiaries who are otherwise entitled to private insurance.

Table 3. Provider Reimbursement.

Type of Reform	Act and Year of Reform	Program Impact Assessment
Reimbursement of hospitals: MANDATORY.	§2173, P.L. 97–35, OBRA 1981	*Restriction on payment:* Repeals Medicare and payment methodology limits hospital reimbursement to costs incurred by efficient and economically administered institutions.

Table 3. Provider Reimbursement.

Type of Reform	Act and Year of Reform	Program Impact Assessment
Reimbursement of hospitals: MANDATORY.	§2173, P.L. 97–35, OBRA 1981	*Increases payment levels:* Provides additional payment to hospitals serving a "dispro-portionate number" of low-income and Medicaid/Medicare beneficiaries. Note: In 1987 (OBRA 1987, §4112), disproportionate share (DSH) facilities were defined and a DSH formula was made mandatory. Under the formula, Medicaid utilization rates must be at least one standard deviation among the mean Medicaid inpatient utilization rate, and the facility's low-income use must be 25%. DSH hospitals must have at least two obstetricians who treat Medicaid patients.
Reimbursement of federally qualified health centers: MANDATORY.	§6404, P.L. 101--239, OBRA 1989; §4704, P.L. 101–508, OBRA 1990	*Increases payment levels:* Requires states to reimburse federally qualified health centers (including all services furnished by or through entities receiving federal PHS Act grants) on a reasonable cost basis, as defined under federal rules, for all FQHC required services and all other ambulatory services under the state Medicaid plan that they furnish.

Table 3. Provider Reimbursement.

Type of Reform	Act and Year of Reform	Program Impact Assessment
Payment for services of Medicaid providers: MANDATORY.	§6402, P.L. 101–239, OBRA 1989	*No additional cost:* Codifies existing federal regulation that requires that payments to Medicaid providers be "sufficient to enlist enough providers so that care and services are available under the plan, at least to the extent that such services are available to the general population."
Payment for obstetrical and pediatric services: MANDATORY.	§6402, P.L. 101–239, OBRA 1989	*No additional cost:* Requires states to submit payment levels and supporting documentation to demonstrate that obstetric and pediatric payment levels are reasonable. Data must show how HMO payments have been adjusted to take the reasonableness requirement into account. Obstetric services include obstetric, family practice (FP), and mid-level services. Pediatric services include pediatrician, FP, and mid-level services. Excludes inpatient and outpatient hospital services and other institutions.
Payment adjustments for hospital services furnished to infants and children under age 6: MANDATORY.	§302, P.L. 100–360, MCCA 1988 and §4604, P.L. 101–508, OBRA 1990	*Increases costs:* Requires states in making payment for inpatient services furnished to young children to include outlier adjustments for stays

Table 3. Provider Reimbursement.

Type of Reform	Act and Year of Reform	Program Impact Assessment
		involving exceptionally long lengths or exceptionally high costs. Also prohibits use of otherwise applicable length of stay or dollar limits. Expands on provision originally enacted under §302 of MCCA 1988 which required coverage of medically necessary inpatient care for infants and payment adjustments for DSH facilities.
Payment for hospice services: MANDATORY.	§6404(c), P.L. 101–239, OBRA 1989	*Increases costs:* Mandates minimum payment levels for hospice services under certain conditions.

Table 4. Federal/State Financing Arrangements.

Type of Reform	Act and Year of Reform	Program Impact Assessment
Reduction in federal Medicaid expenditures: MANDATORY.	§2161, P.L. 97–35, OBRA 1981	*Reduces federal expenditures:* Federal amounts owed to states for permissible expenditures decreased by 3%, 4%, and 4.5% from Fiscal years 1982–84. States may "earn back" reductions through various cost control devices or in the event of high unemployment.
Restriction of federal financial participation (FFP) for high error rates: MANDATORY.	§135, P.L. 97–248, TEFRA 1982	*Reduces federal payments:* Financial penalties imposed for states whose programs

Table 4. Federal/State Financing Arrangements.

Type of Reform	Act and Year of Reform	Program Impact Assessment
		exceed federally established error rate standards. Errors assigned for payment on behalf of ineligible persons or for overpayments but not for denial of coverage of payment in the event of an eligible person or covered service.
Federal financial participation in Medicaid-prescribed drug programs: MANDATORY.	§4401, P.L. 101–508, OBRA 1990	*Increases federal and state spending:* Denial of FFP for state prescription drug programs that do not meet minimum federal requirements including having an approved drug rebate agreement in effect for covered drugs. Minimum federal rebate standards are set. States may impose prior authorization on covered drugs with the exception of new drugs. States may cover certain non-rebate drugs only if they make a finding, and the Secretary concurs, that the drug is essential to the beneficiary's health. States may continue amount, duration, and scope restrictions only if they are consistent with medically accepted indications set by the manufacturer and with safeguards against unnecessary utilization. State maximum allowable costs are prohibited, as are state formularies.

Appendix A

Table 4. Federal/State Financing Arrangements.

Type of Reform	Act and Year of Reform	Program Impact Assessment
		All drugs with rebate agreement must be covered.
Restrictions on federal financial participation in certain state medical assistance expenditures: MANDATORY.	P.L. 102–234, Medicaid Moratorium Amendments of 1991	*Reduces federal expenditures and increases state costs:* Eliminates federal financial participation in certain types of state medical assistance expenditures resulting from non-broad-based provider taxes and contributions. Establishes upper limits, for FFP purposes, on amount of state expenditures resulting from lawful, broad-based provider taxes that qualify for federal contributions. Outlaws all provider donations except bona fide donations. Permits FFP for state Medicaid expenditures resulting from intergovernmental transfers so long as the source of the transfer is not an outlawed tax or donation. Establishes "look-behind" program to assure that tax arrangments do not include "hold harmless" provisions to protect providers against impact of a tax. Sets upper FFP limits on payments to DSH facilities.
Veteran's pension reductions: MANDATORY.	§4410, P.L. 101–508, OBRA 1990	*Increases state costs:* Reduces the pensions of veterans in Title XIX nursing homes, thereby

Table 4. Federal/State Financing Arrangements.

Type of Reform	Act and Year of Reform	Program Impact Assessment
		lowering spend-down liability and increasing Medicaid coverage.
Maintenance of effort with respect to Medicaid coverage: MANDATORY.	§302, P.L. 100–360, MCCA, 1988	*No additional cost:* Prohibits states from reducing AFDC payments below May 1988 levels.

Table 5. State Administration.

Type of Reform	Act and year of Reform	Program Impact Assessment
Freedom of choice waivers: OPTIONAL.	§2175, P.L. 97–35, OBRA 1981	*Either reduces or increases costs:* Permits states to seek waivers of federal "freedom of choice" guarantee, eliminating from the program otherwise qualified Medicaid providers, and requiring beneficiaries to choose among remaining qualified providers. Certain providers excluded and cost efficiency anticipated by reducing unnecessary utilization. However, greater access to care may also increase costs.
Home- and community-based care waivers: OPTIONAL.	§2176, P.L. 97–35, OBRA 1981	*No cost increase:* Persons who otherwise would receive care in institutions may be cared for in community-based settings with expanded services so long as cost of community care does not exceed estimated aggregate cost of state's institutional programs.

Table 5. State Administration.

Type of Reform	Act and year of Reform	Program Impact Assessment
Repeal of EPSDT 1% penalty: MANDATORY.	§2178, P.L. 97–35, OBRA 1981	*No cost impact:* Ceases AFDC federal payment penalty imposed on states that failed to inform, screen, and treat eligible children. Virtually no penalty had actually ever been enforced.
Patient costsharing: BOTH OPTIONAL AND MANDATORY.	§131, P.L. 97–248, TEFRA 1982	*May either increase or reduce costs:* Permits states to impose copayments on certain beneficiaries but exempts children, pregnant women, and persons in long-term care institutions whose only income is a personal needs allowance.
Patient costsharing experiments: MANDATORY.	§131, P.L. 97–248, TEFRA 1982	*No direct cost impact:* Prohibits Secretary from waiving TEFRA costsharing provisions for §1115 experiments unless the experiment tests a unique and previously untested hypothesis, lasts for no more than two years, and either provides for compensation of patients in the event of injury or else is voluntary.
Liens and recoveries: OPTIONAL.	§132, P.L. 97–248, TEFRA 1982	*Reduces expenditures:* States permitted to impose liens on the homes of institutionalized living recipients in certain cases.
Expansion of federally qualified HMOs to include state-qualified HMOs and certain federally funded	§2178, P.L. 97–35, OBRA 1981, and §2364, P.L. 98–369, DEFRA 1984	*Projected to save costs:* Permits states to enroll Medicaid patients in state-qualified HMOs and allows certain federally

Table 5. State Administration.

Type of Reform	Act and year of Reform	Program Impact Assessment
community health centers not previously covered: OPTIONAL.		funded community health centers to be qualified as federal HMOs, depending on their level of federal grant funding and years of operation.
External review of HMOs: MANDATORY.	§9421, P.L. 99–509, OBRA 1986	*May increase costs:* Requires annual external audits of HMOs participating in Medicaid.
Third-party liability: MANDATORY.	§9503, P.L. 99–272, COBRA 1985	*Both increases and reduces state costs:* Requires states to use "cost avoidance" system for collecting third-party liability except in the case of services for pregnant women, EPSDT services for children, and services for which payment owed by an absent parent covered by a medical support order is not made.
Nursing home reform: MANDATORY.	§4211, P.L. 100–203, OBRA 1987	*Increases costs:* Broad revision of standards for certifying and measuring the performance of skilled nursing facilities, rehabilitation institutions, and other long-term care institutions (excluding those for the treatment of mental disease).
Clarification of treatment of educationally related services: MANDATORY.	§411, P.L. 100–360, MCCA 1988	*Increases costs:* Clarifies state obligation to pay for services furnished to children receiving services under Parts B or H of the Individuals with Disabilities Education (IDEA) if they are also services covered under a

Table 5. State Administration.

Type of Reform	Act and year of Reform	Program Impact Assessment
		state Medicaid plan, even if services would be paid through the IDEA system in the case of non-Medicaid–eligible children.
Liberalization of eligibility standards and methodologies for certain categories of Medicaid-eligible persons. Inclusion of state indigent care expenditures in calculating medically needy applicants' spend-down obligations: OPTIONAL.	§303, P.L. 100–360, MCCA 1988	*Increases costs:* Permits states to establish more generous eligibility standards and methodologies for certain classes of non-cash assistance applicants than those used under federal cash assistance programs. Affected classes include poverty-level pregnant women and children, medically needy persons, institutionalized benefi-ciaries, qualified Medi-care beneficiaries, and other optional coverage eligibles.
Required coordination with supplemental food program for women, infants, and children (WIC): MANDATORY.	§6406, P.L. 101–239 OBRA 1989	*Increases and reduces costs:* States required to notify eligible Medicaid recipients of WIC benefits and refer to WIC agency.
Out-stationed enrollment for poverty-level pregnant women and children: MANDATORY.	§4602, P.L. 101–508, OBRA 1990	*Increases costs:* Requires states to provide for out-stationed enrollment of poverty-level pregnant women and children at certain sites, including at minimum, federally qualified health centers and disproportionate share hospitals. States must use forms other than those used to apply

Table 5. State Administration.

Type of Reform	Act and year of Reform	Program Impact Assessment
		for AFDC and must provide for the initial receipt and processing of applications at the out-stationed sites.
Modification of paternity programs: MANDATORY.	§4606, P.L. 101–508, OBRA 1990	*May increase or reduce costs:* Exempts certain pregnant women from having to disclose paternity as a condition of Medicaid eligibility.

INDEX